Specialty Competencies
in School Psychology

Series in Specialty Competencies in Professional Psychology

ROSEMARY FLANAGAN
JEFFREY A. MILLER

Specialty Competencies
in School Psychology

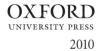

OXFORD
UNIVERSITY PRESS
2010

OXFORD
UNIVERSITY PRESS

Oxford University Press, Inc., publishes works that further
Oxford University's objective of excellence
in research, scholarship, and education.

Oxford New York

Auckland   Cape Town   Dar es Salaam   Hong Kong   Karachi
Kuala Lumpur   Madrid   Melbourne   Mexico City   Nairobi
New Delhi   Shanghai   Taipei   Toronto

With offices in
Argentina   Austria   Brazil   Chile   Czech Republic   France   Greece
Guatemala   Hungary   Italy   Japan Poland   Portugal   Singapore
South Korea   Switzerland   Thailand   Turkey   Ukraine   Vietnam

Published by Oxford University Press, Inc.
198 Madison Avenue, New York, New York 10016
www.oup.com

Oxford is a registered trademark of Oxford University Press

Library of Congress Cataloging-in-Publication data on file
ISBN-13 9780195386325 Paper

9 8 7 6 5 4 3 2 1

Printed in the United States of America
on acid-free paper

ABOUT THE SERIES IN SPECIALTY COMPETENCIES IN PROFESSIONAL PSYCHOLOGY

This series is intended to describe state-of-the-art functional and foundational competencies in professional psychology across extant and emerging specialty areas. Each book in this series provides a guide to best practices across both core and specialty competencies as defined by a given professional psychology specialty.

The impetus for this series was created by various growing movements in professional psychology during the past 15 years. First, as an applied discipline, psychology is increasingly recognizing the unique and distinct nature among a variety of orientations, modalities, and approaches with regard to professional practice. These specialty areas represent distinct ways of practicing one's profession across various domains of activities that are based on distinct bodies of literature and often addressing differing populations or problems. For example, the American Psychological Association (APA) in 1995 established the Commission on the Recognition of Specialties and Proficiencies in Professional Psychology (CRSPPP) in order to define criteria by which a given specialty could be recognized. The Council of Credentialing Organizations in Professional Psychology (CCOPP), an inter-organizational entity, was formed in reaction to the need to establish criteria and principles regarding the types of training programs related to the education, training, and professional development of individuals seeking such specialization. In addition, the Council on Specialties in Professional Psychology (COS) was formed in 1997, independent of APA, to foster communication among the established specialties, in order to offer a unified position to the pubic regarding specialty education and training, credentialing, and practice standards across specialty areas.

Simultaneously, efforts to actually define professional competence regarding psychological practice have also been growing significantly. For example, the APA-sponsored Task Force on Assessment of Competence in Professional Psychology put forth a series of guiding principles for the assessment of competence within professional psychology, based, in part, on a review of competency assessment models developed both within (e.g., Assessment of Competence Workgroup from Competencies Conference—Roberts et al., 2005) and outside (e.g., Accreditation Council for Graduate Medical Education and American Board of Medical Specialties, 2000) the profession of psychology (Kaslow et al., 2007).

Moreover, additional professional organizations in psychology have provided valuable input into this discussion, including various associations primarily interested in the credentialing of professional psychologists, such as the American Board of Professional Psychology (ABPP), the Association of State and Provincial Psychology Boards (ASPBB), and the National Register of Health Service Providers in Psychology. This wide-spread interest and importance of the issue of competency in professional psychology can be especially appreciated given the attention and collaboration afforded to this effort by international groups, including the Canadian Psychological Association and the International Congress on Licensure, Certification, and Credentialing in Professional Psychology.

Each volume in the series is devoted to a specific specialty and provides a definition, description, and development timeline of that specialty, including its essential and characteristic pattern of activities, as well as its distinctive and unique features. Each set of authors, long-term experts and veterans of a given specialty, were asked to describe that specialty along the lines of both functional and foundational competencies. *Functional competencies* are those common practice activities provided at the specialty level of practice that include, for example, the application of its science base, assessment, intervention, consultation, and where relevant, supervision, management, and teaching. *Foundational competencies* represent core knowledge areas which are integrated and cut across all functional competencies to varying degrees, and dependent upon the specialty, in various ways. These include ethical and legal issues, individual and cultural diversity considerations, interpersonal interactions, and professional identification.

Whereas we realize that each specialty is likely to undergo changes in the future, we wanted to establish a baseline of basic knowledge and principles that comprise a specialty highlighting both its commonalities with other areas of professional psychology, as well as its distinctiveness. We look forward to seeing the dynamics of such changes, as well as the emergence of new specialties in the future.

Although "School Psychology" first became recognized as a specialty in professional psychology by CRSPPP in 1998, this area of psychology can be traced back to the late 19th century, where it can be thought to have developed alongside "Clinical Psychology" due to the types of cases seen in Lightner Witmer's Psychological Clinic that opened in 1896. More specifically, as described in chapter 1, clinical cases treated in this clinic included children with learning and behavior problems similar to those seen today by the typical school psychologist. Over the years, this psychology specialty has begun to encompass the science and practice of psychology with regard to a wide range of "learners," including children, youth, and families, as it impacts the schooling or educational process. In this volume, Drs. Flanagan and Miller provide a comprehensive overview of the foundational and functional competencies related to the specialty of school psychology. As the U.S. attempts to reclaim its stature as a leader in education, school psychologists are likely to play a crucial role across multiple tasks and levels. As such, the reader interested in school psychology will find this volume very "educational."

Arthur M. Nezu
Christine Maguth Nezu

References

Kaslow et al. (2007). Guiding principles and recommendations for the assessment of competence. *Professional Psychology: Research and Practice, 38*, 441-451.

Roberts et al. (2005). Fostering a culture shift: Assessment of competence in the education and careers of professional psychologists. *Professional Psychology: Research and Practice, 36*, 355-361.

This work is dedicated to my parents, Angela and Patrick Flanagan, with deep appreciation for their love, support and encouragement. RF

This book is dedicated to my wife Tammy, who has worked tirelessly on behalf of the profession of school psychology and to my son Mason, who is the greatest source of pride in my life. JAM

CONTENTS

PART I

Introduction to
School Psychology

ONE

Definition of School Psychology

What Is School Psychology?

The archival description of school psychology adopted by the Division of School Psychology of the American Psychological Association (APA, 2005) begins by stating: "School Psychology is a general practice and health service provider specialty of professional psychology that is concerned with the science and practice of psychology with children, youth, families; learners of all ages; and the schooling process." This statement indicates that the field of school psychology shares professional interests with clinical and counseling psychology while being broader with regard to its theory and knowledge base in both psychology and education, domains of practice, and research agenda. The National Association of School Psychologists (NASP, 2003) acknowledges on their website (www.nasponline.org) that school psychologists are highly trained in both psychology and education and help youth succeed academically, emotionally, and socially. School psychologists provide a range of assessment, intervention, and preventive services. These services can include evaluations of child and adolescent development, health promotion, and programmatic services for youth, all of which take place within the context of schools, families, and other systems. Intervention is provided for individuals and systems, the primary goal of which is to promote positive learning environments for youth from diverse backgrounds.

History of School Psychology

School psychology (Fagan, 2001) practice has been driven by and is intertwined with its history. In fact, the growth, development, and maturation of school psychology has been a function of developments *outside* the field. These developments include compulsory schooling, the child study movement, and the growth of the special education enterprise (Braden, J., DiMarino-Linnen, & Good, 2001; Fagan & Wise, 2007). Moreover, the choice that psychologists made, to be employees of school systems, may have had the greatest impact on the field because school psychology was subsequently shaped and driven by education (Fagan & Wise, 2007).

School psychology began alongside clinical psychology in Lightner Witmer's Psychological Clinic that opened in 1896. Witmer's description of the types of cases seen in the clinic, including children with learning and behavior problems, is remarkably similar to those typically seen today in school psychology practice (see Fagan, 2000, for a discussion). Those early cases highlighted the importance of understanding the learning needs of low-functioning youth. Other factors contributing to a focus on children's needs were the enactment of laws for compulsory schooling (e.g., Hollingsworth, 1933) coupled with the large numbers of immigrant children who entered U.S. schools in the late 19th and early 20th centuries. Not surprisingly, similar needs regarding low-functioning youth were noted in Europe. In 1905, Binet and Simon developed the first modern test of cognitive ability in France; their purpose was to conduct assessment to determine the needs of exceptionally low-functioning children. Goddard brought the Binet-Simon scale to the United States, and Terman and Merrill, who were based at Stanford University, made some modifications to it in 1916. This test became the Stanford-Binet Intelligence Scale.

By the late 1920s the needs of immigrant children were apparent and led to the development of the Bureau of Child Guidance in New York City. (The bureau operated until the mid 1970s, when the Education for all Handicapped Children Law, PL-94-142, was passed. The requirements of the legislation made the Bureau obsolete). As more needs of youth were identified, the necessity for school psychology training programs emerged. The first training programs appeared at New York University in the 1920s and the University of Pennsylvania in the 1930s; then, in the 1940s, New York and Pennsylvania began to regulate school psychology practice. By the time of the Thayer conference—the conference of the APA school psychology division to determine training standards—in 1954, 20 states and the District of Columbia formally regulated the practice of school psychology (Cutts, 1955, cited in Fagan, 2005). School psychology practice is now regulated in all states (Fagan, 2005). The formal regulation of school psychology is through state departments of education; the first certification acts for school psychology predated licensure of psychologists.

Following World War II, the baby boom resulted in increased demand for psychological services in the schools simply because of the increased numbers of youth. During this same time period, psychology truly became a regulated (licensable) profession, which was most evident in the growth of clinical psychology and the eventual development of doctoral programs to specifically train clinical psychologists. Because practitioner training was essentially generic, clinical psychologists were often able to obtain credentials for school-based practice. Professional psychology grew as a whole, and development of training programs of increased specificity followed. Although the numbers of school psychologists grew, those trained at the subdoctoral level outnumbered those with doctorates. By the late 1960s the need for organization and representation among school psychologists other than APA, which recognized only doctoral-level psychologists, had become evident.

The APA represented school psychologists but only those with doctorates; anyone practicing as a school psychologist at the subdoctoral level was limited to associate membership. Because that limitation was viewed as untenable for some, the National Association of School Psychologists was born in 1969 (See Fagan, 1993, for a discussion). Its growth in membership quickly eclipsed that of APA's Division of School Psychology. Concurrently, for doctoral level school psychology, several developments emerged that further shaped training and practice—namely, the first accreditation of a doctoral school psychology program at the University of Texas at Austin in 1971 by the American Psychological Association (Fagan & Wise, 2007) and the institution of board certification in school psychology by the American Board of Professional Psychology (ABPP) in 1968 (Flanagan, 2004). Only licensed, doctoral-level psychologists are eligible for board certification. These developments made it clear that there was a place for school psychologists who were trained at both the doctoral and subdoctoral levels as professional school psychologists.

Growth in the need for school psychological services and school psychologists continued. An important event in the history of school psychology ensuring its primary practice settings as school was the passage of the Education for all Handicapped Children Act (PL 94-142) in 1975 (Fagan, 2001). The subsequent amendments and revisions to this act have expanded the reach of school psychological services, has reaffirmed the place of school psychologists and their service in schools, and continues to drive practice innovations and trends.

What Are the Professional Boundaries of School Psychology?

The APA (2005) regards school psychology as a general practice specialty and therefore recognizes that the practice activities of school psychologists can be similar to those of other professional psychologists, such as clinical, counseling, and child and adolescent psychologists. School psychology differs from other specialties in professional psychology because there is a focus on applying psychological knowledge and methods to solve problems of schooling and learning (Tharinger, Pryzwansky, & Miller, 2008). The school as a context for development is the primary distinguishing feature of school psychology. Additional defining features are that school psychologists understand the school as an organization that is in a reciprocal relationship with the community, and they are uniquely knowledgeable about the laws and regulations that govern schools and youth with disabilities (Tharinger et al., 2008).

The APA (2005) maintains that school psychologists are trained to provide a range of psychological services in a broad array of settings, although the school setting is primary. Although most school psychologists are employed in schools (NASP, 2003), school psychological services are not limited by setting. School psychological services can include psychological assessment, intervention, prevention, and health promotion as well as program development and evaluation services that emphasize the developmental processes of children and youth within the context of schools, families, and other systems. Interventions may be with individuals or systems. NASP (2003) similarly maintains that school psychologists work to find solutions by using different strategies to address student needs and to improve school and districtwide support systems. Both APA and NASP see school psychologists as working at the individual and system levels to develop and implement programs promoting positive learning environments by training teachers and parents about effective teaching, learning, and behavior management. APA expands this idea further and notes the importance of ecologically valid assessment and program evaluation. These differences parallel some differences in training, as APA accredits doctoral training programs only whereas NASP accredits training at the specialist (i.e., subdoctoral) and doctoral-level school psychology programs. It is important to note, however, that both organizations work to serve all school psychologists; it is the emphasis that differs.

Additional aspects of the functioning of school psychologists include being sensitive to the needs of diverse youth, promoting health development, and collaborating with parents and teachers to further the success of youth.

Technical information, such as test data and theories of development, are often explained to parents, teachers, and youth to promote success. The practice emphasis is more commonly related to school success, although the promotion of successful functioning outside the confines of the school building is also within the purview of school psychologists. The preventive, assessment, consultative, and intervention activities of school psychologists are synthesized and integrative, spanning a range of youth and family needs.

Preventive services can be informational, such as classroom presentations, staff development activities for school-based colleagues, and Parent-Teacher Association meetings. Preventive services can be programmatic; programs may be developed by the school psychologist to address specific issues of concern (NASP, 2003). Follow-up on large group informational activities will often focus on applying the information presented to help small groups or individuals implement recommendations. Collaboration with community agencies may also result in preventive services (NASP, 2003).

Assessment activities vary from brief screenings to determine whether the child's functioning is developmentally on track to psychoeducational assessments to determine whether some form of special education is appropriate. Behavioral assessment is used to determine the nature of the difficulty and develop interventions to improve a youngster's social, emotional, or behavioral functioning. Similar assessment methodologies such as curriculum-based assessment can be applied to instructional environments to facilitate or increase learning. Indeed, assessment spans cognitive, academic, learning, social, and emotional domains. These services are available to all children, irrespective of their (physical) health status.

School psychologists provide various consultative activities, and many of these approaches are now considered traditional in school-based practice: mental health consultation, behavioral consultation, and instructional consultation. Mental health consultation (Caplan, 1995) applies to assistance with child behavior and the adult's feelings about it. Behavioral consultation (e.g., Noell et al., 2005) refers to the assessment of behavior within a context or environment and the collaborative process of developing a plan to address the behavior of concern; there is a research base supporting this process. Instructional consultation (Rosenfield, 1987) refers to assessing the instructional environment and collaboratively developing a plan to increase the effectiveness of instruction. The individuals participating in the consultation process varies by the purpose or type of consultation. For example, behavioral consultation can take place between a school psychologist and a parent, a school psychologist and a teacher, or all three stakeholders may work together to develop a plan. Moreover, the child should be involved as appropriate, given the child's age and the problem of concern. In contrast, instructional consultation typically occurs between teachers and school psychologists. There is a research base to support the different varieties of consultation as practiced by school psychologists.

Consultation might also include parent or teacher conferences, or meetings with a child to discuss a concern; this type of consultation often occurs in conjunction with some other type of school psychological services. School psychologists conduct consultation to promote effective home-school relationships and effective partnerships with the community (APA, 2005; NASP, 2003).

Intervention services include group and individual counseling; the design, implementation, and monitoring of behavioral and instructional plans; and crisis intervention. The provision of psychotherapy by school psychologists is less common. Psychotherapy is more likely to be provided in school-based mental health clinics or independent practice rather than in public schools.

School psychologists also contribute to the knowledge base of the field by conducting research. Even when formal research is not being conducted, the approach to problems is systematic and guided by knowledge of measurement, evaluation, and research principles. Thus, quality assurance and treatment integrity are areas that school psychologists understand and they can assist other school colleagues by sharing their expertise when these skills are needed.

Populations Served

Keeping in mind that everyone (including those who are exceptionally impaired) is expected to attend some form of compulsory education, it is theoretically possible for all youth to have access to school psychologists. While it is not the norm for *all* youth to have been served by a school psychologist, it is possible. The point here is that school psychologists work with a wide range of youth and, in many cases, the school psychologist is the first, if not the only, mental health professional that children and families have contact with. Among the youth served are preschoolers, gifted youth, educationally disabled youth, youth with medical problems, and those whose first language is not English as well as individuals of all ages engaged in structured learning activities.

School psychologists do not limit their client contact to youth. It is not unusual for school psychologists to spend significant amounts of time working with parents, teachers, and other stakeholders to increase the effectiveness of those individuals with students. The broad client base that school psychologists serve is common to practice at the subdoctoral (specialist) and doctoral level. Important to note is that the American Psychological Association (APA) and National Association of School Psychologists (NASP) share common ground yet differ in their conceptualizations of school psychology. For example, while both conceptualizations note the importance of the psychology and education fields, school psychologists are considered professional psychologists by APA. NASP considers school psychologists as being in both the psychology and education fields. It is fair to state that this is in part a function of the breadth and depth of the field.

School psychologists do not limit their practice to the school setting. Compared to all other psychologist specialties—child, clinical, counseling, educational, experimental, forensic, social, and so on—this is the only specialty that derives its name from the place where most school psychologists are professionally located. Although over 83% of school psychologists are employed in public schools (Curtis, Lopez, Batsche, & Smith, 2006), school psychological services are also delivered in preschools, private schools, hospital and clinic settings, independent practice, and university-based (training) clinics. A small percentage (3.5%– 6.5%) of school psychologists serve as faculty in training programs (Curtis et al., 2006; Fagan, 2008); school psychology faculty are commonly known as trainers. Currently there is a shortage of school psychologists and it is troubling that the most severe part of this shortage may be within the faculty ranks. The faculty shortage limits the number of individuals a training program can produce if it is to maintain its accreditation.

What Are the Practice Activities of School Psychologists?

ASSESSMENT

Among the practice activities of school psychologists is the completion of psychoeducational evaluations that include the assessment of an individual's overall developmental cognitive ability and academic achievement, as well as personality and social/emotional functioning. The purpose of these evaluations is for the psychologist to understand students' learning and behavior problems so as to plan interventions. Frequently, assessment is conducted to determine a student's eligibility for special education services; for this, school psychologists also rely on diagnostic/assessment data from other school personnel and integrate these multiple data sources to make appropriate recommendations for youth (APA, 2005). The job function of conducting psychoeducational assessments is in accordance with the

Individuals with Disabilities Education Improvement Act (IDEIA, 2004) and is driven by an educational rather than a psychological classification of disorders such as the *Diagnostic and Statistical Manual of Mental Disorders* (*DSM-IV-TR*; American Psychiatric Association, 2000). Some intervention services provided by school psychologists, such as individual and group counseling, are delivered to meet the mandates of the IDEIA.

CONSULTATION

School psychologists meet with parents, teachers, and other school personnel to review the functioning of youth. This begins the process of collaborative problem solving to assess the concern and plan, develop, and carry out interventions to address instructional and behavioral problems. Consultation, as practiced in contemporary school psychology, tends to be an *indirect service*, meaning that the school psychologist works with the adults who in turn learn to work with the youth in new ways. In ideal circumstances, the indirect service model allows the school psychologist to provide services to many more children. This also means that to be an effective consultant, the school psychologist needs to be knowledgeable about a wide range of child and adolescent concerns across domains. These concerns can span from mild variation of normal development to complex learning, behavioral, medical, and social-emotional problems. School psychologists also facilitate the adjustment and learning of youth who are not native speakers of English. The development and implementation of prevention programs as well as crisis intervention might also be categorized under consultation. Consultation as a direct service includes meeting directly with individuals to do intake interviews, crisis intervention, counseling, or psychotherapy—activities that occur in other practice domains of professional psychology. Consultation in school psychology is often used to address and manage concerns earlier rather than later when they may become chronic.

School Psychology and the Foundational and Functional Competencies

The foundational and functional competencies (e.g., Kaslow, 2004) expected of professional psychologists across practice domains provide one framework from which the contemporary practice of school psychology might be conceptualized. Foundational competencies cover reflective practice, self-assessment, scientific knowledge and methods, relationships, diversity, and ethical and legal standards. Functional competencies include the knowledge, skills, and values needed to perform the work of a psychologist; these include assessment, diagnosis, case conceptualization, intervention, consultation, research and evaluation, supervision, teaching, management, and administration (Rodolfa et al., 2005).

Specifically for school psychology, these competencies include practice skills in assessment, interpersonal relations with a broad range of clients, counseling and intervention skills as well as ethical and respectful practice. The knowledge base of school psychologists includes multiple theoretical perspectives and empirical findings in the areas of education, learning, normal and abnormal development, social psychology, statistics, psychometrics, and research procedures. Despite the breadth and depth of knowledge and skills conceptualized by the functional and foundational competencies, the uniqueness of the knowledge base, as described by Lambert (1986) as necessary for an effective professional school psychologist, is not thoroughly captured. Lambert maintained that it is the knowledge base above all that distinguishes school psychology from other practice specialties for youth. It was Lambert's belief that the doctoral school psychologist must have a solid knowledge base of research and theory to be an effective consultant; her approach to training emphasized the application of knowledge to solve problems over the professional skills that are called upon when solving problems. This notion is also consistent with ethical standards regarding competence (Knapp & VandeCreek, 2006). The current movement toward a competency-based approach in professional psychology considers the knowledge base and professional skills to be equally important components of functioning. Nevertheless, school psychologists have a unique knowledge base compared to the closely aligned specialties of clinical, counseling, and child/adolescent psychology. The most skillful doctoral school psychologists would have a highly developed knowledge base and superior practitioner skills; this combination is very desirable and is evaluated in the examination for the American Board of Professional Psychology (ABPP) diploma in school psychology.

Kaslow et al. (2007) have outlined 15 principles to guide the assessment of competence of professional psychologists. Important to these principles is the notion that this assessment by colleagues is an ongoing process, occurring in a developmental context. Among the parameters of competence are practice skills, knowledge, interpersonal skills, sensitivity to diversity, ethical practice, and the ability to be a reflective practitioner. The assessment of competence should utilize multiple methods. Assessment is only part of the picture. Maintaining competence in new skills and practices is an ongoing activity for professional psychologists that should incorporate consultation and supervision with experts (Barnett, Doll, Younggren , & Rubin, 2007).

Training and Credentialing of School Psychologists

Note that the necessary and sufficient credential for school-based practice is subdoctoral and is issued by state departments of education. The majority of school psychologists are credentialed at this level only. School psychologists who are not employed in schools typically need additional credentials to meet regulatory requirements.

If a school psychologist who possesses a doctoral degree desires, he or she may seek generic licensure as a psychologist though the state board for psychology. Some states offer licensure for school psychologists at the subdoctoral level. This credential is often in addition to the credential needed for school-based employment/practice. Regulation varies by state, typically in statute, as do the parameters of practice. Some school psychologists may be able to meet requirements to become a mental health counselor or marriage and family therapist by completing additional coursework and internships. These credentials are also regulated in statute and are open to individuals trained at the subdoctoral level.

Credentials for the independent practice of psychology—similar to those for other psychologists, such as clinical psychologists—are available at the doctoral level and are issued by state boards of psychology. School psychologists who are also credentialed by their respective state boards of psychology may also be recognized as health service providers by the National Register of Health Service Providers in Psychology and are eligible to pursue board certification through the American Board of Professional Psychology. Board certification through the ABPP is the highest credential available to professional psychologists.

TWO

Conceptual, Theoretical, and Scientific Foundations of School Psychology

The fields of counseling, clinical, and school psychology have at times been claimed to lack distinct focus as differentiated specialties of professional psychology (Matarazzo, 1987; Minke & Brown, 1996). On the contrary, we argue that school psychology, in both purpose and conceptual foundation, is a specialty that is highly differentiated from either counseling or clinical psychology. In this chapter we first discuss the purpose of school psychology as being significantly different from that of other professional psychology specialties. This purpose provides the field with a range of opportunities while at the same time laying a clear parameter outlining the boundaries of the specialty. Next, we examine the conceptual basis of the specialty, showing it as the necessary glue that holds together the profession's judgments about the application of theory and empirical data to the practice of school psychology. We show that school psychology has a clear purpose distinct from other areas of professional psychology, a signature conceptual foundation, and a theoretically integrated basis that is informed by the empirical literature for the practice of school psychology, and that these features define the distinct specialty of school psychology within professional psychology.

Purpose of School Psychology

Keith (1998) makes a compelling argument that school psychology needs to identify a central *purpose* that provides the field with a common frame for practice. Borrowing from Trachtman (1981), Keith eloquently concludes that "the purpose of school psychology is to enable children, youth, and adults to profit from education" (p. 14). This is a very powerful statement that is sufficiently focused to provide a proprietary purpose to the activities of school

psychologists while being sufficiently inclusive not to tie the hands of inno-
vators of school psychology practice. Specifically, Keith says that this purpose
provides an answer not to *what* we do but rather to *why* we do it. Kamphaus
(1998) raises an important point that dovetails with this purpose, that is, education is not limited to public schools. Rather, education encompasses public
and private elementary and secondary education, higher education, corporate training, military training, and informal education. School psychologists
should be the "go to" professionals for services to enable individuals to profit
from education of all kinds. This is an important distinction: the specialty of
school psychology is not bound by the physical location of a school building;
rather, it is bound by the activity of facilitating education. Indeed, school psychology should not limit itself to the school building because it is inevitable
that the practice of education will increasingly be conducted in online, cyber
environments (Allen & Seaman, 2008; Christensen, Johnson, & Horn, 2008).
As we discuss, this frame of purpose provides a freeing yet delimiting role for
school psychology practice. So, to conduct assessment with a child in a public
school is to enable a child to profit from elementary or secondary education.
To consult with a corporate training office on best practices to train employees
on a new software program is to enable adults to profit from their educational
experience (Kamphaus, 1998). To conduct statewide program evaluation of a
new mathematics curriculum is to enable policy makers to make decisions so
that children may profit from their mathematics education.

The purpose of school psychology is to facilitate education in all environments, not just in schools.

Keith (1998) suggests that there is a finite universe
of activities or roles subsumed under the purpose of
enabling individuals to profit from education. This
universe of roles can be used as the framework in
which the field makes decisions about what roles and
functions should be added to the activities of school
psychologists, what activities may be outside the purpose of school psychology, and what activities school psychologists may be *missing* as essential to
helping individuals profit from education. The next section provides coverage of the conceptual foundation of school psychology and the set of theoretical perspectives that school psychologists turn to in the effort to enable
children, youth, and adults to profit from education.

A Model for School Psychology Practice

CONCEPTUAL FOUNDATIONS OF SCHOOL PSYCHOLOGY

School psychologists are asked to deal with *wicked problems*. This is not to say
the problems are evil or malicious but that they are so complex that solutions

are often elusive. Rittel and Webber (1973) defined wicked problems in their seminal paper on policy and planning. Basically, a wicked problem is one that has incomplete, contradictory, and changing parameters in a context of complex interdependencies. It is critical to understand that school psychologists are primarily working with wicked problems. The danger is when school psychologists think they are working with routine problems that are completely parameterized in an isolated context. This is dangerous because it encourages a culture of complacency that may fail to reveal the real complexities in even the most mundane, routine referrals. In the following we discuss the conceptual framework that is used by school psychologist adherents of broad-ranging approaches ranging from systems theory to applied behavior analysis to bring down the barriers and build the bridges to allow individuals to profit from education.

Rittel and Webber (1973) argued that a single scientific base is insufficient to account for the complex problems of society. This is truer today than it was in 1973. Ramo (2009) describes our society in the 21st century as a complex, international society that is impervious to simple prevention tactics. Our society is so interdependent and complex that all problems are unlikely to be anticipated and it is therefore necessary to implement prevention tactics that minimize the impact of a crisis. That is, crises and problems will occur; what should be planned for is sufficient resiliency in the system to recover from the crisis or problem. This is true for the world, country, state, school district, school, classroom, teacher, and student. These complex, hierarchical systems are in constant interaction and transaction and they are organic in that they cannot be parameterized in a linear way. Rather, the parameters are nonlinear and often very difficult to anticipate. Thus, for school psychology to be able to serve the learners in this context, the conceptual frame must have the capacity to account for these hierarchical complexities (Bronfenbrenner, 1979). Therefore, it has been argued that the core conceptual base of school psychology is an *ecological-transactional model* of human behavior (Gutkin & Reynolds, 2009). This model is then used to organize information from broad theoretical and empirical bases for the practice of school psychology.

The ecological aspect of this model has been offered as a core model of behavior in school psychology in a variety of publications (e.g., Meyers & Nastasi, 1999; Reynolds, Gutkin, Elliott, & Witt, 1984; Woody, LaVoie, & Epps, 1992). The ecological model organizes environmental factors that influence behavior from proximal to distal and states that these factors interact in complex ways (Bronfenbrenner, 1979).

The practice of school psychology is based on the *ecological-transactional model* of human behavior.

Bandura's (1978) notion of reciprocal determinism—in which the person, the behaviors, and the environment reciprocally influence each other—has been used to describe the complex interactions among ecological factors (Reynolds et al., 1984). A more modern approach to explaining these interactions, it could be argued, is that they are *transactional*, and the child's behavior and development are influenced by the exchanges between other developing individuals and a changing environment (Mercer & DeRosier, 2008). The school psychologist's conceptualization of transactions within the child's ecology is informed by the primary theories that undergird school psychology training.

The specialty of school psychology has evolved from a general perception that the problems reside within the child, consistent with a medical model, to a perception that the child's *psychology* is important to the extent that it is in the context of an ecological milieu that reciprocally impacts the child. Unlike a clinical or counseling psychologist who may take multiple contexts and multiple modalities of functioning into consideration, the school psychologist is *part of* the milieu and interacts with the child's transactions in situ. This provides both the strength of the school psychologist's understanding of the problem and the weakness of not being completely objective. That is, it is much easier to make a clinical diagnosis from the distal vantage of a clinic or private practice office because all of the myriad confounding information inherent in ecological transactions is minimized through self and/or parent report. The school psychologist, on the other hand, knows the school environment, the classroom teacher, the special subject teachers (e.g., art, music) , the community, the child's parents and likely grandparents, the curriculum, the child's peers, the school leadership, the district, the economic situation, the child's siblings, legal environment, and so on. The school psychologist can and must take all of these elements into consideration for case conceptualization. Further, he or she must consider these same variables for group (e.g., classroom) and system problem solving in educational settings. Even what may appear to be the most discrete intervention—for example, learning basic multiplication facts via the taped-problems intervention (McCallum, Skinner, Turner, & Saecker, 2006)—requires consideration of the classroom teacher, available technology, children in the classroom, treatment integrity, and school policy regarding augmenting curricula. To make any intervention work in the context of a school setting is complex. The primary contexts of this ecological milieu are the child's psychology comprised of cognitive, behavioral, emotional, and social functioning; the school setting; the family setting; and the community. The model is transactional in that these different contexts influence each other. This is further complicated because these transactions impact a dynamically changing child moving through various stages of human development. From this perspective, it is apparent that school psychologists perform highly complex roles and require specialized training to be able to appropriately manage this volume of contexts and interactions. This necessity to *understand* and *engage in* the ecological-transactional model is a unique feature of the specialty of school psychology that differentiates it from other specialties and necessitates a broad theoretical knowledge base.

Theoretical Foundations in School Psychology

The theoretical foundations central to school psychology are developmental psychology (including developmental psychopathology),learning theory (applied behavioral analysis and cognitive psychology), psychological measurement theory, personality and social psychology, biological psychology, and organizational and systems theory. Table 2.1 provides example peer-reviewed publications in school psychology representing each of these theoretical domains. When school psychology students are introduced to this range of theories in their first graduate course on the role and function of school psychology, they are unanimously overwhelmed. After the course of training, however, it is gratifying to see them practice competently across such a vast range of theoretical domains while always considering the ecological-transactional conception of school psychology practice. They are able to become a part of the system of education and bring to bear a broad range of knowledge to help individuals and groups profit from education. Thus, it is notable that the practice of school psychology is highly *theoretically integrated*, but grounded in the ecological experience of the students.

CHILD DEVELOPMENTAL THEORY

Whether working with an individual child or a group of children, or whether working directly or indirectly with children, the school psychologist must always take into consideration normal and abnormal child development. This is a core consideration for assessment, intervention, and consultation. Child development covers a broad range of child characteristics that develop over time from before birth

Theoretical Foundations of School Psychology

- Developmental psychology
- Learning theory
- Psychological measurement theory
- Personality and social psychology
- Biological psychology
- Organizational and systems theory

TABLE 2.1 **Example Articles Representing Theoretical Domains in School Psychology**

THEORY	EXAMPLE SCHOOL PSYCHOLOGY PUBLICATIONS	
Learning Theory	Bradshaw, C. P., Koth, C. W., & Bevans, K. B. (2008). The impact of school-wide positive behavioral interventions and supports (PBIS) on the organizational health of elementary schools. *School Psychology Quarterly, 23*, 462–473.	Bellini, S., Akullian, J., & Hopf. (2007). Increasing social engagement in young children with autism spectrum disorders using video self-modeling. *School Psychology Review, 36*, 80–90.
Developmental Psychology	Schwartz, E., & Davis, A. S. (2006). Reactive attachment disorder: Implications for school readiness and school functioning. *Psychology in the Schools, 43*, 471–479.	Hojnoski, R. L., & Missall, K. N. (2006). Addressing school readiness: Expanding school psychology in early education. *School Psychology Review, 35*, 602–614.
Personality & Social Psychology	Aalsma, M. C., Lapsley, D. K., & Flannery, D. J. (2006). Personal fables, narcissism, and adolescent adjustment. *Psychology in the Schools, 43*, 481–491.	Andreou, E. (2006). Social preference, perceived popularity and social intelligence: Relations to overt and relational aggression. *School Psychology International, 27*, 339–351.
Biological Psychology	Phelps, L. (2008). Tourette's disorder: Genetic update, neurological correlates, and evidence-based interventions. *School Psychology Quarterly, 23*, 282–289.	Volker, M. A., & Lopata, C. (2008). Autism: A review of biological bases, assessment, and intervention. *School Psychology Quarterly, 23*, 258–270.
Psychological Measurement Theory	Hintze, J. M. (2005). Psychometrics of direct observation. *School Psychology Review, 34*, 507–519.	Thompson, T., Sharp, J., & Alexander, J. (2008). Assessing the psychometric properties of a scenario-based measure of achievement guilt and shame. *Educational Psychology, 28*, 373–395.
Organizational and Systems Theory	Bonner, M., Koch, T., & Langmeyer, D. (2004). Organizational theory applied to school reform. *School Psychology International, 25*, 455–471.	Adelman, H. S., & Taylor, L. (2007). Systemic change for school improvement. *Journal of Educational & Psychological Consultation, 17*(1), 55–77.

to adulthood. Specific areas that form the school psychologist's knowledge base include physical (including brain), social, emotional, personality, and cognitive development. In addition, school psychologists must be fluent in abnormal development as described by developmental psychopathology, neurodevelopmental disorders, and physical disability.

LEARNING THEORY

Learning theory in education comprises diverse approaches to how individuals learn. This is of course critical to the school psychologist because many of the referral concerns involve individuals who are having difficulty learning. Teaching and learning are the primary business of schools. The primary learning theory approaches taught are behavioral learning theory and cognitive learning theory. Behavioral learning theory is highly empirical and assumes that learning occurs through reinforcement in the environment that is contiguous with the behavior. There are a variety of techniques that comprise behavioral learning theory including positive and negative reinforcement, shaping, errorless learning, response cost, and so on. Cognitive learning theory on the other hand has a significant interaction between theory and empirical evidence. It is concerned with explaining learning from a brain-based perspective and explaining how the mind is organized to produce thought (Anderson, 2004).

PSYCHOLOGICAL MEASUREMENT THEORY

Measurement theory in psychology is particularly critical to school psychologists as they apply the theory in a number of different ways during their practice. Most obvious is the use of psychological and educational tests developed using measurement theory. School psychologists are taught that it is not enough to administer a test in a standardized manner; rather, it is necessary to understand how the test was constructed and the theoretical underpinnings of the constructs. For example, one cannot assume generalization of the norms from a test to an individual being assessed. The individual may be older or younger than the norm group or there may be a significant underrepresentation of the child's ethnicity in the norm group. School psychologists will have to adopt into their practice new versions of tests as well as tests of new constructs over their life span. As such, school psychologists must be able to review new tests in a critical manner before including them in an assessment battery. Further, the school psychologist must be able to judge the validity of the constructs purported to be measured by the test. It is widely known that the Cattell-Horn-Carroll (CHC; Phelps, McGrew, Knopik, & Ford, 2005) model of human intelligence is applied in the design and interpretation of modern tests of cognitive functioning. It is impressive that this model has such widespread adoption on these tests. However, there are other constructs of cognitive functioning that are only peripherally covered by the CHC model, such as working memory. It is insufficient to apply just the CHC model for the design and interpretation of memory and learning tests as the model is not comprehensive enough to account for the highly developed models of working memory. Rather, the school psychologist should expect to see Baddeley's (2003) theory of working memory used as a primary organizing theory to suggest that the test is theoretically sound. This level of analysis is critical to protecting clients and ensuring that psychological evaluations are as valid as possible. It can be seen that measurement theory provides windows not only into the technical aspects of tests' validity and reliability but also into the theoretical foundations of the constructs tests purport to measure.

PERSONALITY AND SOCIAL PSYCHOLOGY

Personality and social psychology, along with biological psychology (see next section), are required components of APA accredited training programs in professional psychology. It should therefore be no surprise that they are included as a part of the theoretical foundations of school psychology. However, personality and social psychology are not just covered in passing but are critical to the practice of school psychology. First, a knowledge of personality psychology is necessary for a psychologist to be able to assess the developing personalities of children with emotional problems and to promote positive emotional growth. Also, as children approach the age of considering the world of work, the psychologist should be able to provide some guidance about a child's personality disposition for various career options. This expectation to plan for the world of work is mandated by the federal special education law IDEA. Second, school psychologists work in the social milieu of learning environments, particularly in public school settings. Social psychology theory is necessary to make sense of children's behavior in large and small groups, to help make school policy decisions, to understand group behavior in team meetings with school faculty members, and to understand what drives decision making across a variety of social and academic situations.

BIOLOGICAL PSYCHOLOGY

School psychologists have needed to gain an understanding of biological psychology for more reasons than because it is considered a core competency in professional psychology. In particular to school psychologists, biological psychology is applied because many of the disorders that impair a person's ability to benefit from the learning environment have a biological basis, most noticeably attention-deficit/hyperactivity disorder (Barkley, 1997). In addition, low-incidence disorders have a biological basis: multiple sclerosis, asthma, Down syndrome, and cystic fibrosis, to name a few. School psychologists assess the impact of the disorders on functioning and must take into consideration the physiological causes and limitations that are associated with these disorders. Among the learning problems that have a biological basis, learning disabilities are by far the most prevalent. Although school psychologists have long assessed cognitive functioning in relation to learning disabilities, increasingly they are recognizing that learning disabilities are brain-based disorders (Shaywitz, 2003) and this has driven them to make an intentional adoption of neuropsychological assessment and interpretation (Hale & Fiorello, 2004). Although school psychologists are being trained in neuropsychology in a limited way at the nondoctoral level, it is clear that doctoral-level school psychologists are qualified due to their extensive training in assessment to acquire the postdoctoral specialization of neuropsychology.

ORGANIZATIONAL SYSTEMS THEORY

As consultants and agents of change in large and small institutions of teaching and learning, school psychologists need to learn the processes of organizational change and the structural organization of a school district underneath a superintendent to be able to make meaningful change in schools (cf. Bolman & Deal, 2003). The school psychologist must learn how to roll out schoolwide and sometimes districtwide initiatives to improve learning. On a broader level, school psychologists take part in preparing organizations for change (Merrell, Ervin, & Gimpel, 2006) in part by bringing data-based problem solving to a wide range of problems and constituencies in the school. School psychologists who apply principles of organizational systems theory become some of the most trusted leaders in a school district because they approach problems with the added benefit of understanding individual human behavior.

Inquiry Methods in School Psychology

School psychologists become practitioners in a variety of settings and many of them become trainers in university settings with the primary responsibility of generating new knowledge in the field. They must be trained consumers of research. Nevertheless, the inquiry methods used by each set of professional school psychologists differ in large part because of set-ting. University researchers in school psychology often rely on larger scale nomothetic research methodologies and small *n* or single-subject studies to advance knowledge. On the other hand, the practitioner typically embraces a single-subject approach consonant with the local clinical scientist (Stricker & Trierweiler, 1995) model of practice. Finally, both often engage in pro-gram evaluation, an increasingly important role for school psychologists. Table 2.2 shows published articles in school psychology representing the inquiry methods described in this section.

Inquiry Methods Used by School Psychologists

- Nomothetic — the study of groups of individuals

- Ideographic — small or single-subject studies

- Quantitative — research that relies on statistical tests of null hypotheses

- Qualitative — research that relies on opinions and beliefs rather than statistical data

CONSUMERS OF RESEARCH

School psychologists are trained to be lifelong learn-ers, and in that role they are expected to keep up with developments in the professional knowledge base. Practicing school psychologists and univer-sity trainers do so through a variety of means. By virtue of membership in professional school psy-chology organizations, they have access to research that is synthesized and summarized in articles in professional newsletters and magazines such as the *Communiqué* and the APA *Monitor*. Also, member-ship in these professional organizations gives them access to research journals such as the *School Psy-chology Quarterly* and *School Psychology Review*. For a school psychologist to go beyond these sources, it is helpful to have access to full-text database compilations of current and past research such as *PsycArticles*. Both major professional organizations in school psychology (APA and NASP) are working to make access to such valuable resources affordable to practitioners. An approach applied in med-icine, but less so in school psychology, is the publication of practice parame-ters endorsed by major professional organizations that provide authoritative syntheses of the empirically based diagnostic procedures and interventions associated with various types of problems.

NOMOTHETIC APPROACHES TO RESEARCH

Researchers in school psychology utilize experimental designs and quasi-experimental designs to build the knowledge base in professional school psy-chology. Nomothetic approaches typically rely on quantitative data analysis approaches such as statistics. Statistical methods applied include regression analysis, ANOVA, structural equation modeling, and hierarchical linear

TABLE 2.2 Example Articles of Inquiry Methods Used by School Psychologists

METHODOLOGY	EXAMPLE SCHOOL PSYCHOLOGY PUBLICATIONS	
ANOVA/ Regression	Oliver, R., & Williams, R. L. (2006). Performance patterns of high, medium, and low performers during and following a reward versus non-reward contingency phase. *School Psychology Quarterly, 21,* 119–147 (ANOVA)	Ostrov, J. M., & Crick, N. R. (2007). Forms and functions of aggression during early childhood: A short-term longitudinal study. *School Psychology Review, 36,* 22–43. (Regression)
Structural Equation Modeling	McMahon, S. D., Parnes, A. L., Keys, C. B., & Viola, J. J. (2008). School belonging among low-income urban youth with disabilities: Testing a theoretical model. *Psychology in the Schools, 45,* 387–401.	Taub, G. E., Keith, T. Z., Floyd, R. G., & McGrew, K. S. (2008). Effects of general and broad cognitive abilities on mathematics achievement. *School Psychology Quarterly, 23,* 197–198.
Hierarchical Linear Modeling	Murdock, T. B., Beauchamp, A. S., & Hinton, A. M. (2008). Predictors of cheating and cheating attributions: Does classroom context influence cheating and blame for cheating? *European Journal of Psychology of Education, 23,* 477–492.	Volpe, R. J., DuPaul, G. J., Jitendra, A. K., & Tresco, K. E. (2009). Consultation-based academic interventions for children with attention deficit hyperactivity disorder: Effects on reading and mathematics outcomes at 1-year follow up. *School Psychology Review, 38,* 5–13.
Psychometric Methods	Pelletier, J., Collett, B., & Gimpel, G. (2006). Assessment of disruptive behaviors in preschoolers: Psychometric properties of the Disruptive Behavior Disorders Rating Scale and School Situations Questionnaire. *Journal of Psychoeducational Assessment, 24,* 3–18.	Suldo, S. M., & Shaffer, E. J. (2007). Evaluation of the self-efficacy questionnaire for children in two samples of American adolescents. *Journal of Psychoeducational Assessment, 25,* 341–355.
Single-Subject Design	Treptow, M. A., Burns, M. K. & McComas, J. J. (2007). Reading at the frustration, instructional, and independent levels: The effects on students' reading comprehension and time on task. *School Psychology Review, 36,* 159–166.	Cates, G. L. (2005). Effects of peer versus computer-assisted drills on mathematics response rates. *Psychology in the Schools, 42,* 637–646.

(continued)

TABLE 2.2 **Example Articles of Inquiry Methods Used by School Psychologists — *Continued***

METHODOLOGY	EXAMPLE SCHOOL PSYCHOLOGY PUBLICATIONS	
Meta-analysis	Merrell, K. W., Gueldner, B. A., & Ross, S. W. (2008). How effective are school bullying intervention programs? A meta-analysis of intervention research. *School Psychology Quarterly, 23,* 26–42.	Burns, M. K., & Wagner, D. A. (2008). Determining an effective intervention within a brief experimental analysis for reading: A meta-analytic review. *School Psychology Review, 37,* 126–138.
Qualitative Methodology	Kennedy, E. K., Frederickson, N., & Monsen, J. (2008). Do educational psychologists "walk the talk" when consulting? *Educational Psychology in Practice, 24,* 169–187.	Leech, N. L., & Onwuegbuzie, A. J. (2008). Qualitative data analysis: A compendium of techniques and a framework for selection for school psychology research and beyond. *School Psychology Quarterly, 23,* 587–604.

modeling. These techniques are used to answer a variety of questions ranging from treatment effectiveness to descriptive analyses of problem profiles. In addition to these approaches, meta-analyses are commonly applied to synthesize the research in a specific area. Another, obviously larger scale approach is psychometric methodology, often used by test development companies; however, many individual researchers and research teams work to apply classical and modern test theory to develop new psychological tests and evaluate existing tests. Methodologies employed include classical reliability and validity approaches based on correlation, multitrait-multimethod, and advanced Rasch modeling and other latent trait approaches.

IDEOGRAPHIC METHODOLOGIES

As previously indicated, both practitioners and university researchers utilize small *n* or single-subject design methodologies. Single-subject designs allow researchers to examine interventions by looking at a small number of participants at baseline and then measuring them over time after the intervention has been implemented. Often multiple baselines as well as reversal designs, in which treatment is removed temporarily, are used to control for threats to the internal validity of the study. Single-subject designs provide the majority of evidence cited for empirically based interventions in school psychology.

Action research is often applied in clinical settings to answer specific questions raised by administration and staff. Action research is usually less concerned with generalizability than research designed to have a broad impact. Approaches used in action research include single-subject methods involving a child or two in the classroom or broader survey studies of a school building or even a school district. The analytic method tends to not be statistical but relies on the observation of patterns in the data.

Both of these approaches are consonant with the local clinical scientist model of training and practice (Stricker & Trierweiler, 1995). The local clinical scientist model argues that findings that are relevant to a particular local context may or may not be relevant to other contexts and the only way to find out is to publish local findings so that practitioners in other settings may also benefit from knowing the findings. The research methodology intentionally does not aim at generalizability but works to solve problems in the local milieu; when such results are published, however, other school psychologists will have an opportunity to determine whether the intervention fits their local situation. Hughes, Kaufman, and Miller (2010) recently commented that the local clinical scientist model shows great promise for bridging the research-to-practice gap by encouraging more practitioners to engage in empirical inquiry and to do so with university researchers in an intentional way.

QUALITATIVE METHODS

Increasingly, qualitative methodologies are being utilized in school psychology. Such methods include ethnography and phenomenology (Leech & Onwuegbuzie, 2008). These methods are particularly well suited for organizational and systems change processes. For example, working to close the achievement gap requires a genuine understanding of students, parents, and teachers in a system, and qualitative methods have been helpful in clarifying patterns and nuances involved in trying to resolve such major problems.

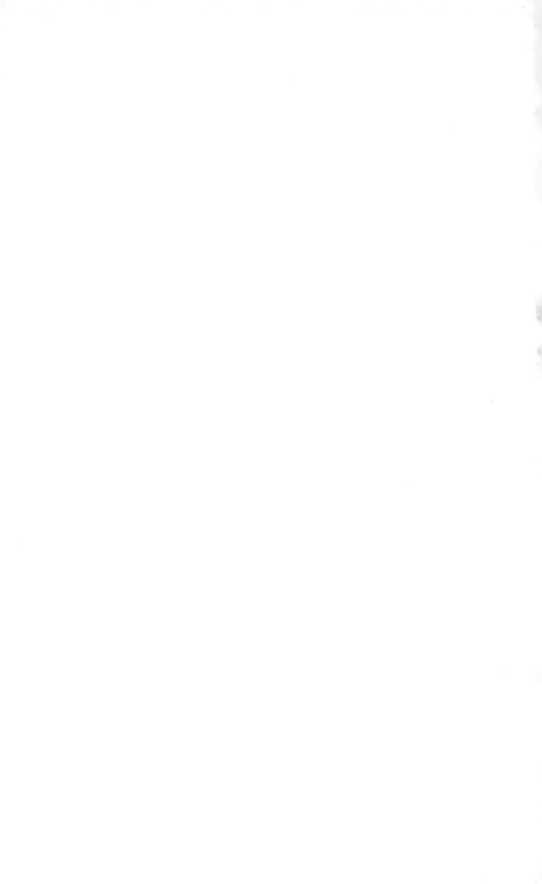

PART II

Functional Competency—
Assessment

THREE

Assessment Strategies I

Assessment in general and psychoeducational assessment in particular are central roles for school psychologists (Fagan & Wise, 2007). Despite intense debate within the field about the relevance of psychoeducational assessment, at the end of the day it is the primary role of school psychologists (Hosp & Reschly, 2002; Wnek, Klein, & Bracken, 2008) and has provided individualized education program teams with the necessary data to understand why a child is struggling with learning and make recommendations about how to help. Indeed, it is the primary purpose of psychoeducational assessment to provide recommendations (Merrell et al., 2006). School psychologists who employ an ecological-transactional approach to psychoeducational assessment provide recommendations that include a broad range of causes for learning problems. This is in sharp contrast to the medical model in which the problem is assumed to be within the child (Reynolds, Gutkin, Elliot, & Witt, 1984). Rather, the typical approach of the school psychologist should be to consider the strengths and weaknesses of the child in the context of his or her developmental history and social and educational milieu. These factors provide the richness of context necessary to make psychoeducational test data germane to a problem-solving approach.

The purpose of this chapter is to first outline the typical approach to psychoeducational assessment used by school psychologists and discuss the implications of this approach to case conceptualization. Next, there is a discussion of current measures commonly used in psychoeducational assessment across the domains of cognitive, academic achievement, and social-emotional functioning, including

Psychoeducational assessment is the primary role of school psychologists.

projective or performance-based measures. In addition to a discussion of tests and test batteries, we cover behavioral observation, interview, performance-based measures, adaptive functioning, and neuropsychological assessment. The chapter concludes with a discussion of current controversies about the strengths and weaknesses of psychoeducational assessment.

Approaches to Psychoeducational Assessment

Sattler (2008) wrote a seminal work on the psychoeducational assessment of children in his book entitled *Assessment of Children,* now in its fifth edition. He conceptualizes psychoeducational assessment as having four pillars: norm-referenced testing, interviews, observations, and informal assessment procedures. Norm-referenced testing is the topic of the first section of this chapter and includes tests that have been developed using psychometric theory and that compares individuals being assessed to a clearly defined norm group. That is, typical performance is defined by the normative sample and individuals being assessed are compared to that sample to determine whether they are functioning within the average, less than average, or above average range of functioning. Typically, standardized scores and percentiles that are scaled to the norm group's performance are used to describe individual functioning. Interviews, in the context of child evaluations, can be either structured or unstructured and are typically conducted with the learner, the learner's teacher, and significant others as needed. Observations occur in naturalistic settings as well as in assessment sessions and provide valuable data about the learner's functioning in the milieu as well as information about approaches to problem solving. Finally, informal assessment procedures include nonstandardized assessment procedures such as passage reading, solving math problems, or play-based assessment. These pillars of assessment form the data sources that are used to achieve assessment outcomes such as decisions on entitlement to special education, diagnoses, clinical impressions of strengths and weaknesses, and recommendations. These outcomes are most commonly achieved when the school psychologist frames assessment as a problem-solving process (Merrell et al., 2006).

Four Pillars of Psychoeducational Assessment

- Norm-referenced testing — comparing to the normative sample
- Interviews — can be structured or unstructured
- Observations — occur in naturalistic settings
- Informal assessment — includes nonstandardized assessment procedures

Assessment in the Problem-Solving Process

Merrell and colleagues (2006) provide a succinct overview of psychoeducational assessment as a problem-solving process. The process starts by clarifying the referral question through record review, interview, and observational data. This is necessary because referral questions sometimes assume that a disorder exists (for example, "the child needs an ADHD evaluation") or are sufficiently general that the referral question doesn't serve to narrow the problem space (for example, "the child doesn't behave at school"). Thus, referral questions must be filtered by the school psychologist based on clinical experience in relation to preliminary data collection. It should be noted here that not all referrals for comprehensive evaluation should be accepted. This is particularly the case when prereferral intervention has not been implemented with integrity or at all (Schrank et al., 2004). This process of prereferral intervention is commonly codified in school districts as response-to-intervention, which is described in greater depth in chapter 4.

Steps to Psychoeducational Assessment

1. Clarify referral question
2. Form a hypothesis
3. Choose fixed or flexible battery
4. Conduct assessment
5. Synthesize data
6. Formulate recommendations and interventions

Once the referral question is sufficiently clarified, the school psychologist forms one or more hypotheses about potential reasons for the referral concern (Hale & Fiorello, 2004; Kamphaus, 2009). These hypotheses narrow the scope of the assessment to relevant instruments and procedures. At this point, it is instructive to discuss the differences between fixed and flexible assessment batteries. As we show, the flexible battery approach is more amenable to hypothesis testing in assessment.

The *fixed battery* means that the school psychologist uses the same set of assessment procedures for all referral concerns. This has the advantages of allowing the school psychologist to be very well versed in the tests used and to develop "internal" norms, examiner expectations about performance on tests, about how individuals in general perform on these tests. Using an unimaginative fixed battery approach has resulted in school psychology having a public relations problem because it seemed to some that all referrals resulted in the child taking an intelligence test and an achievement test as a fixed battery. The fixed battery in general, and the limited fixed battery of a "WISC and WIAT," suggests there are a priori assumptions about the child's problems, dismisses the ecological-transactional nature of most problems, and points to an assumption that all necessary data are subsumed by the fixed battery. A *flexible battery* approach, on the other hand, usually includes a standard set of assessment instruments with additional instruments introduced based on the hypotheses of the professional school psychologist. Further, the school psychologist can add additional tests based on the responses to previous tests, which is consonant with a problem-solving approach. This approach is viewed as more economical in terms of assessment time, but also more comprehensive in that a wider range of relevant psychological processes is assessed.

To use the flexible battery approach effectively, the school psychologist must be well versed in multiple measures. He or she must also understand the strengths and limitations of instruments. Indeed, it is important to select assessment instruments according to the constructs measured and how the constructs are operationalized, the intended use of the instrument, and its psychometric properties. No one instrument will perform better than others in *all* situations. In fact, how the youngster may respond to the instrument can be a key consideration because a poor response will likely compromise the validity of the data. For example, referred preschoolers often have speech articulation issues; and school psychologists are expected to obtain a measure of cognitive ability. With the availability of well-constructed measures that limit the need for spoken responses, it behooves the school psychologist to utilize tools that limit this threat to validity. Thus, it is important to be familiar with multiple measures of cognitive ability, academic achievement, learning skills, social-emotional functioning, and so forth in order to craft a flexible battery that provides quality data in an efficient manner.

Once the assessment procedures have been completed, the data need to be synthesized to determine whether the hypotheses are supported. To make the process of integrating and interpreting assessment data manageable, a stepwise process based on data from each pillar of assessment can be followed. The process proceeds from divergent to convergent thinking within each assessment modality, pillars of assessment and domains within each pillar, and then proceeds to integrating all assessment modalities (Hughes, T.L. & Morine, 2005). For example, start with the direct observation results. The task first is to (1) find patterns and (2) to identify inconsistencies within the observation notes. Initial attempts to formulate hypotheses about consistencies and discrepancies should be divergent—broad and open-minded considerations of all possible explanations are consistent with the problem-solving approach. This process is repeated with the interview data, behavioral rating data, and norm-referenced test results. After each modality has been examined, two assessment modalities are compared. The school psychologist asks, are the consistencies and discrepancies within the two modalities the same or different? Are there any similar interpretations that account for assessment data across the two modalities? What revisions to the previously determined interpretations are necessary to accommodate the data from both modalities? This process continues until all assessment data have been examined together. From this process, convergence will emerge in which similar causes of learning problems are identified and corroborated across different assessment modalities.

Conclusion about the nature of the problem then leads the school psychologist to formulate recommendations and interventions. The analysis of data should have included examination of prereferral interventions and what in those interventions worked and did not work. It goes without saying that the same interventions should not be recommended without some explanation of how to implement them differently for them to be effective. Recommendations in a written report are often organized around referral concerns such as reading or inattention. These recommendations can also be organized around cognitive or personality features such as working memory or impulsiveness (Mather & Jaffe, 2002). Specific intervention recommendations will be covered in chapter 6.

Test Construction and Fair Testing

School psychologists are familiar with and apply the principles outlined in the *Standards for Educational and Psychological Testing* (American Educational Research Association [AERA], American Psychological Association [APA], National Council on Measurement in Education [NCME], 1999). This book describes, among other things, the standards for test construction and fairness in testing. Each of these is briefly discussed later in the chapter.

TEST CONSTRUCTION

School psychologists are responsible for using tests of the highest psychometric quality possible, with the recognition that test results include error and professional judgment is necessary to interpret them properly. Since many school psychologists are involved in test construction, they also are held to the requirements discussed in *Standards*.

Validity   A fundamental consideration is the validity of the test. *Validity* "refers to the degree to which evidence and theory support the interpretations of test scores entailed by proposed uses of tests" (AERA, APA, & NCME, 1999, p. 9). It can be seen that validity is more than whether the test measures what it purports to measure. Rather, consideration must be given to the intended purpose of the test and the linkage between the usefulness of the test to guide decisions for that purpose (Messick, 1995). Validity evidence can be garnered from examination of the content of the test (content validity), comparison of test scores with external criteria (criterion-related validity), and through examination of its internal structure (construct validity). Messick (1995) has argued that validity evidence should take into consideration more explicitly the use of particular tests and recommends that construct validity evidence be expanded to include content, substantive, structural, generalizable, external, and consequential aspects. He further argues that by recognizing that validity evidence is not a property of the test itself but rather is a property of the interaction between the test, its users, respondents, and the purposes of the test, validity can apply to all assessment including performance assessment such as portfolios that do not necessarily have standardized stimuli.

Reliability   Test users are responsible for examining the reliability of an assessment procedure. *Reliability* describes the consistency of a measure, the degree to which a test measures the same way each time it is used. Further, it is an indication of the amount of measurement error expected in the use of a test for a particular group of individuals; higher reliability indicates lower measurement error. Thus, reliability is not a property of the test but a description of the reliability of scores for a group being analyzed (Thompson, 2003). Therefore, it is important to consider the norm group of a test when using a test for a particular child. A test applied to individuals outside the normative sample may not result in stable test scores for those individuals. For example, a test primarily designed for youth in schools may not be as reliable if used with youth in incarcerated settings. Reliability can be estimated using classical test theory by correlating the same test given at two different times (test-retest reliability), comparing two different but equivalent forms of a test (alternate forms reliability), or examining the consistency of the items within the test (internal consistency reliability). Reliability coefficients range from 0 to 1.0 with values closer to 1 indicating better reliability or more consistency in test scores. Error in measurement is indicated by the standard error of measurement. As the standard error of measurement increases (indicating more error in test scores), the reliability coefficient decreases.

Test Construction   The *Standards* recommends four stages of test development. First is the statement of the purpose of the test that includes defining the constructs or domains that will be assessed by the test. The definition of the construct or domains of a test should be empirically supported, but even so, the construct definition is idiosyncratic to the test developer. For example, a test may be said to measure depression. However, if the test is developed from a cognitive-behavioral perspective it may not be valid for a psychiatric evaluation that conceives depression as being largely biological. Second, the specifications of the test need to be delineated. Specifications include, for example, whether it will be a norm-referenced or criterion-referenced test, what age range the test will be used for, and how scores will be reported. The third stage is to develop test items, field test, revise items, and develop scoring guidelines. This process should include examination of the validity and reliability of the test as well as determination of bias. Last, the final version of the test is assembled including the development of documentation so that end users can administer, score, and interpret the test properly.

Four Stages of Test Development

1. State purpose of test

2. Outline specifics of test

3. Develop test items and scoring guidelines

4. Assemble final version of test

FAIRNESS

Fairness in psychological assessment is not a perfectly defined term but rather a notion that the process of assessment will advance social goals of equity and equality of opportunity. It is instructive to reflect on Stephen Jay Gould's (1981) comment in *The Mismeasure of Man*, "The misuse of mental tests is not inherent in the idea of testing itself. It arises primarily from two fallacies, eagerly (so it seems) endorsed by those who wish to use tests for the maintenance of social ranks and distinctions: reification and hereditarianism" (p. 155). Thus, a well constructed, unbiased test is likely not the cause of unfair decisions; rather, these rest with the test user.

Standards provides four views of fairness that should be considered for ethical and fair test construction and use. First is fairness as a lack of bias, which means the test itself is relatively free of bias. Bias, unlike fairness, is a technical term that means "different meanings for scores earned by members of different identifiable subgroups" (AERA, APA, & NCME, 1999, p. 74). There are numerous sources of bias, methods for detecting bias, and approaches to reducing bias that are beyond the scope of this chapter (see Reynolds & Lowe, 2009, for a comprehensive review). The second consideration regarding fairness is equitable treatment in the testing process. All assessment should be conducted according to the test developer's instructions and in a relatively stress free, comfortable environment. When such conditions are afforded differentially to different groups, there is a threat of bias.

Standards recommends that all test takers be given "just treatment" in terms of familiarity with the test procedures, testing conditions, and reporting of test scores. In cases in which accommodations are necessary for individuals with particular disabilities or language differences, such accommodations are detailed in the written summary of the test results. Third is fairness with regard to equity in outcomes of testing. It is well known that there are differences in average levels of performance on some constructs across different racial, ethnic, or gender groups (AERA, APA, & NCME, 1999; Reynolds & Lowe, 2009). These differences have been shown to not be a form of bias and there is no expectation that scores will be equal across subgroups. Rather, the intent of this fairness consideration is that individuals from different subgroups with equal standing on the construct being measured will earn comparable scores on the test. The final consideration has to do with achievement and equality in the opportunity to learn. Similar to the notion of *curriculum bias*, it would be unfair to withhold an opportunity based on test results if the individual did not have an opportunity to learn the information assessed by the test. For example, preventing a student from graduating who did not pass a graduation exam because the student did not have an opportunity to learn the material would be unfair.

Four Views of Fairness in Testing

1. Fairness as lack of bias
2. Fairness as equitable treatment in the testing process
3. Fairness in equality of outcomes of testing
4. Fairness as opportunity to learn

Taken together, high-quality test construction and fair test use allow the school psychologist to gather important and useful data for psychoeducational assessments. In the absence of these standards, the contribution of psychoeducational assessment to the purpose of enabling individuals to profit from learning is compromised. Although these matters of psychological testing may be self-evident, there are recent instances in which there are questions about the adequate implementation of these standards. As one example, there is increased scrutiny on curriculum-based assessment that forms the basis of the response-to-intervention movement for children with learning disabilities (Ardoin, 2006; Ardoin & Christ, 2008; Reynolds & Shaywitz, 2009). Such examples remind every school psychologist to remain vigilant about the standards of psychological and educational assessment.

Cognitive Assessment

Cognitive assessment has its roots in the measurement of individual differences and intelligence testing. Historically, interest in assessing individual differences predates modern psychology. More than 3,000 years ago the Chinese measured individual differences to assign roles in civil service. Since that time efforts have been made to assess intelligence and cognitive functioning explicitly (Kamphaus, 2009), but it was not until Alfred Binet and Theodore Simon developed the first intelligence test to assess individuals with mental retardation (Gould, 1981) that the modern age of cognitive assessment began. In the United States, Lewis Terman in 1916 adapted the Binet-Simon tests and dubbed the battery the Stanford-Binet. Now in its fifth edition, the Stanford-Binet Intelligence Scales is one of the primary measures of cognitive functioning used by school psychologists. Although the first, the Stanford-Binet does not hold the top spot for frequency of use; the Wechsler scales have that distinction.

Wechsler developed his first intelligence test in 1939 called the Wechsler-Bellevue Intelligence Scale, which was later revised to be the first of many Wechsler scales called the Wechsler Intelligence Scale for Children (Wechsler, 1949) and the Wechsler Adult Intelligence Scale (WAIS; Wechsler, 1955). From these beginnings the WAIS has been revised four times, the Wechsler Intelligence Scale for Children is in its fourth edition, and the Wechsler Preschool and Primary Scale of Intelligence is now in its third edition. The Wechsler intelligence scales became the primary procedures for school psychologists in the 1960s and 1970s. This was codified by the passage of PL 94-142, Education for All Handicapped Children Act, in 1975 that functionally required the use of intelligence tests to assess the large numbers of children suspected of having learning disabilities.

The Stanford-Binet and Wechsler scales of intelligence are the primary measures of cognitive functioning used by school psychologists

This trend of assessment has continued, as indicated by a survey of school psychologist members of the National Association of School Psychologists (NASP) conducted by Hosp and Reschly (2002). Data gathered in 1997 indicated that school psychologists spent about 22 hours per week engaged in assessment-related activities, which was about three times as much time spent in the next most frequent activity, intervention. With regard to intellectual assessment, respondents reported administering about 15 intellectual/ability measures per month, about the same number of projective measures administered and second to behavior rating scales (~17 per month). Assessment subsumes a large amount of the school psychologist's time and of that time a large portion includes cognitive assessment.

Significant debate surrounds the use of intelligence tests for a number of reasons. Further, recent changes to federal special education law may impact the frequency of intelligence/ability measures used by school psychologists.

Before talking about the debate it is important to consider the rhetoric. School psychologists have debated whether these test batteries measure a unidimensional general construct of full-scale intelligence, known as *g*, or multidimensional cognitive abilities (Kamphaus, 2009; Miller, D.C., 2007; Sattler, 2001). As Hale, Fiorello, Kavanagh, Hoeppner, and Gaither (2001) point out, this difference is really a matter of what is entered first into a regression equation. When full-scale IQ is entered first, the subscales that are used to compute the full-scale score do not register as significant. This is an obvious statistical principle of shared variance. However, when Hale and colleagues (2001) enter the subscales into regression equations first, the full-scale IQ score does not register as significant. Thus, truly multidimensional scales of cognitive ability get labeled "intelligence" tests, implying a single score, and are relegated as not useful to helping children with learning problems (e.g., Reschly, 1997). The rich information that comes from modern tests of cognitive ability have formed the basis for scientific breakthroughs in the underlying problems of reading difficulties, and the treatment of these underlying cognitive problems has resulted in improvements in reading (e.g., phonological awareness) (Shaywitz, 2003). In part through this process of vilifying measures of cognitive ability by labeling them unidimensional intelligence tests, the federal special education law was changed to include an untested approach to entitlement decisions known as *response-to-intervention (RTI)*. Response-to-intervention will be discussed elsewhere in this book, but it is important to recognize that although the federal law has changed to provide options with regard to processes for identifying individuals with learning disabilities, most school psychologists continue to conduct a comprehensive evaluation after a learner has failed to respond to intervention and before qualifying the individual for special education (Reynolds & Shaywitz, 2009; Schrank, Miller, J.A., Caterino, & Desrochers, 2006).

Theoretical Basis of Cognitive Ability Assessment

The field of school psychology is moving from the notion of a general (*g*) factor (Spearman, 1904) known as intelligence to a multiple factors notion of component cognitive abilities (Carroll, 1993) as central to the assessment process. Wechsler's often cited definition of intelligence, the ability to adapt to the environment (Sattler, 2001), seems dated in the face of broad cognitive abilities that have profiles of strengths and weaknesses for every individual and that characterize people as individuals. The multidimensional nature of cognitive functioning has been debated for years starting in the mid-1900s with Cattell's (1941) two-factor model of crystallized and fluid intelligence.

The two-factor model was revised in the 1960s (Horn & Cattell, 1966) and became a dominant approach, along with a general factor, of interpreting intelligence tests. The major breakthrough in the theory of cognitive abilities came when Carroll (1993) examined about 400 different factor analyses and defined the *Three Stratum Theory* that Kamphaus (2009) describes as the "most important unifying theory currently available" (p. 235). Currently, this theory is called the *Cattell-Horn-Carroll Theory (CHC theory)* and includes 10 broad stratum factors and over 70 narrow abilities (McGrew & Flanagan, 1998) (see sidebar).

Subsets of these factors have been shown to be measured by most modern tests of cognitive ability (Phelps, McGrew, Knopik, & Ford, 2005) and tests such as the Wechsler Intelligence Scale for Children, Fourth Edition, have downplayed the interpretation of full scale IQ or *g* in favor of interpretation of index scores of broad stratum factors.

The 10 Broad Stratum Factors of the Cattell-Horn-Carroll Theory

- crystallized intelligence (Gc)
- fluid intelligence (Gf)
- quantitative reasoning (Gq)
- reading and writing ability (Grw)
- short-term memory (Gsm)
- long-term storage and retrieval (Glr)
- visual processing (Gv)
- auditory processing (Ga)
- processing speed (Gs)
- decision/reaction time/ speed (Gt)

Cognitive Ability Tests Used by School Psychologists

Historically, only a handful of well-normed tests of cognitive ability were in common use: the Stanford-Binet and the Wechsler. Although the Woodcock-Johnson Tests of Cognitive Abilities has been available for thirty years it only recently has become popular. Indications are that use of the Woodcock-Johnson Tests of Cognitive Ability-Third Edition (WJ COG III) is rising (Merrell et al., 2006); this has to do the with the general acceptance of the CHC theory and the fact that the WJ III COG assesses the most CHC factors of any available cognitive abilities test. Table 3.1 lists the current versions of major cognitive abilities tests used by school psychologists as well as the major composite scores provided by each.

Normative Measures of Academic Achievement

The assessment of academic achievement is typically conducted in two ways: standardized, norm-referenced measures of academic skills and criterion-referenced, curriculum-based assessment (Merrell et al., 2006). This section focuses on norm-referenced assessment; curriculum-based

TABLE 3.1 **Tests of Cognitive Ability Used by School Psychologists**

TEST	COMPOSITE SCORES	AGE RANGE
Wechsler Preschool and Primary Scale of Intelligence—III	1. Verbal IQ (VIQ) 2. Performance IQ (PIQ) 3. Processing Speed Quotient (PSQ) 4. General Language Composite (GLC) 5. Full Scale IQ (FSIQ)	2:6–7:3 years
Wechsler Intelligence Scale for Children—IV	1. Verbal Comprehension Index (VCI) 2. Perceptual Reasoning Index (PRI) 3. Working Memory Index (WMI) 4. Processing Speed Index (PSI) 5. Full Scale IQ (FSIQ)	6–16 years
Wechsler Adult Intelligence Scale—IV	1. Verbal Comprehension Index (VCI) 2. Working Memory Index (WMI) 3. Perceptual Organization Index (POI) 4. Processing Speed Index (PSI) 5. Full Scale IQ (FSIQ)	16–89 years
Woodcock-Johnson Tests of Cognitive Abilities—III	Scales: 1. Verbal Ability Scale 2. Thinking Ability Scale 3. Cognitive Efficiency Scale 4. Supplemental Scale 5. Intra-Cognitive Discrepancies Scale 6. Predicted Achievement Scale 7. General Intellectual Ability (GIA) Gf-Gc Composites: 1. Comprehension-Knowledge 2. Long-Term Retrieval 3. Visual Processing 4. Auditory Processing 5. Fluid Reasoning 6. Processing Speed 7. Short-Term Memory	2–90+ years
Stanford-Binet Intelligence Scales—V	Factor Indexes: 1. Fluid Reasoning 2. Knowledge 3. Quantitative Reasoning 4. Visual-Spatial Processing 5. Working Memory IQ Scores: 1. Nonverbal IQ 2. Verbal IQ 3. Full Scale IQ	2–89+ years

TEST	COMPOSITE SCORES	AGE RANGE
Kaufman Assessment Battery for Children — II	Indexes: 1. Mental Processing Index 2. Fluid-Crystallized Index 3. Nonverbal Index 4. Full Scale IQ (FSIQ) Scales: 1. Sequential Processing/Short-Term Memory 2. Simultaneous Processing/Visual Processing 3. Planning Ability/Fluid Reasoning 4. Learning Ability/Long-Term Storage and Retrieval 5. Knowledge/Crystallized Ability	3–18 years
Cognitive Assessment System	1. Planning Scale 2. Attention Scale 3. Simultaneous Processing Scale 4. Successive Processing Scale 5. Full Scale IQ (FSIQ)	5–17 years
Reynolds Intellectual Assessment Scales	1. Verbal Intelligence Index 2. Nonverbal Intelligence Index 3. Composite Memory Index	3–93 years
Universal Nonverbal Intelligence Test	1. Memory Scale 2. Reasoning Scale 3. Symbolic Scale 4. Nonsymbolic Scale 5. Full Scale IQ	5–17 years

assessment (CBA) is covered in chapter 4. Standardized achievement tests assess the core areas of academic achievement such as reading, writing, and arithmetic. Such assessment batteries tend to be designed for use across a wide age range through employing basal and ceiling levels to identify questions that are appropriate for specific age or grade levels. The tests included on these assessment batteries often are organized around the areas of specific learning disability described in IDEA. Thus, there are measures of basic reading, reading comprehension, reading fluency, mathematics computation, applied mathematics, written expression, oral expression, and listening comprehension. It is notable that in the current revision of IDEA the only fluency construct added was reading fluency. Nevertheless, test batteries such as the Woodcock-Johnson Tests of Achievement-Third Edition (WJ ACH III) include fluency measures for not only reading but also mathematics

Academic achievement can be measured through either norm-referenced assessment or curriculum-based assessment.

and writing. Areas such as general knowledge or academic knowledge that cover science and social studies are sometimes included in the test battery (e.g., academic knowledge on the WJ ACH III), but these are rarely used for academic intervention planning because they lack the breadth of content necessary to apply to a science or social studies curriculum. Table 3.2 provides a listing of several common test batteries of academic skills.

Another set of standardized achievement tests includes single-subject tests used to assess a single academic area in more depth and with a broader range of stimulus activities. For example, the *Key Math-Third Edition* (Connolly, 2007) provides coverage of a full range of math skills such as basic concepts, operations, and problem-solving applications across several subtests and with many more questions than would be seen on a typical math test

TABLE 3.2 **Tests of Academic Achievement Used by School Psychologists**

TEST	COMPOSITE SCORES	AGE RANGE
Wechsler Individual Achievement Test—II	1. Reading 2. Mathematics 3. Written Language 4. Oral Language	4–19 years
Woodcock-Johnson Tests of Achievement—III	1. Oral Language 2. Brief Achievement 3. Total Achievement 4. Broad Reading 5. Broad Math 6. Broad Written Language 7. Brief Reading 8. Brief Math 9. Math Calculation Skills 10. Brief Writing 11. Written Expression 12. Academic Skills 13. Academic Fluency 14. Academic Apps	2–90+ years
Kaufman Tests of Educational Achievement—II	1. Reading Composite 2. Math Composite 3. Written Language Composite 4. Oral Language Composite 5. Comprehensive Achievement Composite	4–25 years

in a multi-subject achievement battery. These single-subject test batteries are not used as frequently as multi-subject achievement batteries by school psychologists, but they tend to be used for follow-up assessment when a specific area of academic performance is identified as less well developed from the multi-subject battery.

According to Hosp and Reschly (2002), school psychologists administer about 12 achievement tests per month, making them obviously one of the major techniques used in the specialty of school psychology. Their frequency of use does not reach that of cognitive ability or behavioral rating scales, probably because school psychologists practicing in schools are not the only individuals to administer standardized achievement tests. Often special education teachers are trained to administer achievement tests and do so to monitor progress as well as provide the achievement data for the special education evaluation and reevaluation processes. Regardless, school psychologists are primarily responsible for interpreting and integrating achievement test information as part of the comprehensive psychological assessment.

Social-Emotional and Personality Assessment

Social-emotional, or personality assessment, is an important component of psychoeducational evaluations. In addition to its role as part of the comprehensive evaluation required to determine a student's eligibility for special education, there are other important uses for the data. The data can be used to assist in determining whether psychopathology is in evidence; they may also be used to allow the school psychologist to describe the child and his or her functioning. This description of the child may be used to understand the child's needs, strengths, and limitations. Social-emotional evaluations in school psychological practice often extend beyond the detection of psychopathology, as subclinical issues often negatively impact school functioning and consequently merit attention and intervention.

For example, the social-emotional needs, strengths, and limitations of a child can shed information based on an apparent academic problem that persists despite intact cognitive ability and commensurate scores on standardized achievement tests. Does the child have a deficient self-image? Is the child poorly motivated to succeed? Is the child preoccupied with worries or other negative emotions? This information may help the school psychologist understand what upsets a child, how the child processes or understands social situations, and how the child views people and his or her relationships with others by providing a basis for further assessment that includes the nature of the child's social problem solving. This understanding can provide direction to intervention planning and development. Important to note is that assessment data do not *directly* translate into interventions; rather, the school psychologist must use the assessment data as a point of departure and plan and develop an intervention from scratch or select a commercially available intervention appropriate to the situation (e.g., Shure, 1992a, 1992b, 1992c).

The methods and instruments used to conduct a social emotional evaluation include observations, interviews, questionnaires, and projective, or performance-based (Dana, 2007; Teglasi, 1998) measures of personality.

BEHAVIORAL OBSERVATIONS

A common method used to gather information about a child's behavior and functioning is to observe a child's behavior. The school psychologist will select settings or circumstances within which to observe the child going about his or her usual routines. The setting or circumstances selected will typically relate to the referral question. Important is to focus on observing and gathering facts to conduct a functional assessment. The observed behaviors may be considered within a behavior analytic ABC framework in which "A" is the antecedent, "B" is the behavior, and "C" is the consequence (e.g., Kazdin, 2001). Miller, J.A., Tansy, and Hughes (1998) have conceptualized the overall process of functional assessment as containing two steps: (1) hypotheses are generated about the antecedents and consequences of the behavior, and (2) these are tested systematically.

ABC Model of Behavior

A = Antecedent

B = Behavior

C = Consequence

Although behavior analytic methods are common in school psychology practice, these are not the only methodology, nor is the observational process limited to this methodology. It is important to observe the child and his or her interaction with the context. It is important to gather data of sufficient quality to allow determination of whether a change in context might be a reasonable intervention for a particular child in particular situation. It is important to observe the child's strengths as well as weaknesses and to observe the conditions under which the child's behavior is desirable and when it is not. Essential to this process is an initial emphasis on gathering facts, prior to any hypothesizing or data interpretation. The observation can be structured in a number of ways. Both the type of data sought and the eventual interpretations will be a function of the theoretical orientation of the school psychologist. There are techniques, however, that are more popular among school psychologists whose theoretical orientation is behavioral or cognitive/behavioral. Event recording

(Miller, L. K., 1975) involves noting the particular event each time it occurs. Data may also be recorded by frequency. For purposes of a psychoeducational evaluation, however, the most useful observations may come from taking a running record of the child's behavior for 20–30 minutes. When collected with considerable detail and high accuracy, a great deal of data can be gathered that may be richly presented in context. The reliability and validity of observations are a function of both the observer and the consistency of the child being observed (Miller, L. K., 1975). Reliability and validity could be increased by conducting multiple observations using multiple raters. A less complicated alternative would be the use of commercially available observation forms, such as the Structured Observation System (SOS) of the Behavior Assessment System for Children, Second edition (BASC-2; Reynolds & Kamphaus, 2004). This utilizes time-sampling procedures and provides operational definitions of the behavior to be observed on the form, thereby increasing the reliability and validity of observations. A limitation is that the observation emphasizes certain behaviors only.

INTERVIEWS

The interview method is popular in professional psychology, transcending theoretical orientation (Sattler, 1998). The questions used and the latitude that the interviewer has in formulating questions can vary from open-ended, to semistructured to highly structured. In professional practice, the type and manner of questioning selected will often be a function of the type of information desired as well as the age and cognitive ability of the child. The psychometric properties of the interview data obtained are a function of the type of interview question (open-ended, semi structured, or structured), how forthcoming the child (or adult) is when responding, the ability of the interviewer to know when to question further and when not to, and the interviewer's attention to detail (Cohen & Swerdlik, 2005). The type, quality, and amount of data may also be a function of the rapport between the interviewer and the child. A major strength of the method is that the extent of questioning in any given area can be adjusted as needed during the interview. The interviewer also has the benefit of observing the affect of the child when responding and can note changes in affect that appear prompted by particular questions/topics. A good interviewer can efficiently obtain the contextual and situational information that is essential for data interpretation.

School psychologists should be flexible when interviewing youngsters. Some young children might not understand what is requested of them or may simply be ill at ease responding to an adult in a novel situation. Other young

Types of Interviews
- Open-ended—uses questions that require more than one- or two-word responses
- Semistructured—a flexible approach, allowing new questions to be brought up as a result of what the interviewee says
- Structured—has a formalized, limited set of questions

children may thoroughly enjoy the attention from an adult and reveal considerable information. Interviewers, however, must be skilled and attentive to detail, as a verbose young child is not likely to provide the information in any sort of systematic or organized manner. Moreover, one can be verbose and not provide substantive information. Latency-age children and adolescents will typically understand what is expected of them and the need for thoroughness and attention to detail on the part of the interviewer, yet the cooperation with the interviewer and the process may be limited because they understandably do not wish to reveal information. Important to remember is that youth are not self-referred and may not agree that there is a problem in the first place, making it difficult at times for the interviewer to establish rapport (DiGiuseppe, Linscott, & Jilton, 1995) and obtain the desired information. Yet even the observation that the child is not forthcoming in the interview situation can yield relevant information, depending on the reason for the psychological evaluation.

Despite the pitfalls and limitations of interviewing, this is a powerful way to obtain information from youngsters. It is also important to interview adults such as parents and teachers when evaluating a child; the perspectives of others are invaluable, provide contextual information, and allow for assessment of the environment. Assessing the environment allows one to consider the possibility that despite concerns about the child, the key target for intervention is the environment (or someone in it). Because interview data are subject to technical limitations and distortion, it is important to corroborate the findings. Sources of corroborating data include multiple individuals in an authority relationship with the child, test data, questionnaires, school records, and observational data.

When evaluating a child, it is important to interview parents and teachers as well.

SELF-REPORTS AND BEHAVIOR RATING SCALES

Questionnaires are important assessment tools. Over the past 25 years, many new instruments that are well standardized and validated have become available. The statistical methods used to analyze data and develop norms have become more sophisticated, and questionnaires have stronger psychometric properties. Although these devices are generally used for assessment and problem identification, they might prove useful for progress monitoring under controlled circumstances.

Questionnaires take several forms and can assess single constructs and the associated subconstructs (e.g., Kovacs, 1992) or can be omnibus devices of varying breadth that assess both strengths and weaknesses. Popular are sets of questionnaires that are *omnibus measures* of functioning. These permit multiple raters to comment on the child's strengths and weaknesses (e.g., Reynolds & Kamphaus, 2004). These sets of questionnaires commonly contain a self-report form completed by the child, a parent rating scale, and a teacher rating scale. Both parents and multiple teachers could complete the forms; the data obtained from multiple adult informants is clearly helpful in assessing the context and the adults' view of the child as well as the response of adults to the child's behavior and functioning. This allows the school psychologist to determine whether the significant adults in the child's world are in agreement (this is often not the situation) about the referral concerns. These data can clarify whether the difficulty is more generalized as opposed to being related to one individual or one setting. The youngster's self-report allows for an additional perspective, which can be examined within the context of the ratings provided by adults. Limitations of this method include the length of the measures and, for some respondents, the reading level needed to respond to the questionnaires. Some instruments are available in audiotaped versions (e.g. Reynolds & Kamphaus, 2004) to obviate reading difficulty among respondents.

Also useful are questionnaires that assess single constructs and the associated subconstructs, such as depression (e.g., Kovacs, 1992). In general, these questionnaires are briefer than omnibus measures. Uses include examining a construct in greater or different depth as compared to an omnibus measure so as to generate supplemental data that can broaden the description of the youngster's functioning or allow the interviewer to examine a particular construct in depth from the outset, as suggested by the referral question. Other examples of such questionnaires assess anxiety (Reynolds & Richmond, 2008) and self-concept (Piers, Harris, & Herzberg, 2002).

Professional practice requires that the assessment be tailored to specifically answer the referral question. Thus, school psychologists demonstrating advanced competency will not always use the same set of instruments for all children, although it is appropriate to prefer some instruments over others. An effective assessment is one that integrates the data to arrive at a unique description of the child, which then allows the professional school psychologist to develop recommendations. The integration of test data is discussed elsewhere (Flanagan, Costantino, Cardalda, & Costantino, 2007;

Individual questionnaires can be used to assess single constructs while sets of questionnaires are often used to assess both strengths and weaknesses. These sets typically contain a self-report form for the child, a parent rating scale, and a teacher rating scale.

Riccio & Rodriquez, 2007). An overview of instruments useful in school psychology practice follows.

Behavior Assessment System for Children (BASC)　The Behavior Assessment System for Children, second edition (BASC-2; Reynolds & Kamphaus, 2004) is an extremely popular instrument among school psychologists and will be discussed as a case in point. The BASC-2 was empirically developed according to a factorial model and assesses psychopathology, school and learning-related difficulties, and social adaptive skills for preschoolers through college students. The form and domains assessed vary by age group and rater. Important is that the constructs are operationalized consistently across the forms and the age span of youth. This is useful in schools because youth served by special education are reevaluated periodically, and is useful in other settings/practice situations as well. The parent and teacher forms assess numerous identical constructs; the self-report of personality is needed to provide complementary information. Because the BASC was developed to meet the requirements of special education regulations (Flanagan, 1995), a companion observation form (for frequency and event recording) and developmental history (demographic and background information) is also available. Extensive data are available on BASC-2 to guide practice. The BASC-2 is useful as a screening device and as a measure that provides in-depth information about a child.

Other Multiple Informant Sets of Questionnaires　The Achenbach Empirical System of Behavior and Affect Assessment (AESBA; Achenbach & Rescorla, 2003), the Personality Inventory for Children (PIC; Lachar & Wirt, 2001) and the Personality Inventory for Youth (PIY; Lachar & Gruber, 1994), and the Conners Comprehensive Behavior Scales (Conners, 2007) are other examples of questionnaires developed to be an omnibus evaluation of behavior and affect. Multiple raters are accommodated; the exact forms and scales can vary by the age of the youngster. Each set of questionnaires has features that make it unique; there are similarities and differences in reasons for development, the actual questionnaire development and psychometric properties, and the content of the questionnaires. Each questionnaire set has strengths and weaknesses; practitioners need to be able to understand the technical information in the test manuals to make a fully informed choice of which instrument to use. Doing so is an important part of functional competency as a professional psychologist. Nevertheless, all of these instruments can prove useful in school psychology practice in and out of the schools. It is desirable for practitioners to be open to using different instruments as well as to broadening their assessment repertoire by being skilled with multiple measures of the most commonly assessed constructs, such as tendencies to anxiety and depression.

PERFORMANCE-BASED MEASURES OF PERSONALITY/ SOCIAL-EMOTIONAL FUNCTIONING

Performance-based measures of personality (Dana, 2007; Teglasi, 1998) allow for examination and observation of an individual's functioning while completing a task. Tasks involve sizing up a pictured stimulus, about which the youngster is asked to tell a story that addresses who the characters might be, what led up to the presented scenario, what is presently occurring, what the characters might be thinking and feeling, and how the story turns out. A series of stimulus cards are presented that elicit projection (Frank, 1939), which is a process by which the individual identifies with a pictured stimulus and in so doing, reveals information about himself or herself. The information is not necessarily information that the child wishes to reveal, nor is it necessarily in the child's awareness. Narrative measures used in school psychology for these purposes are the TEMAS (Costantino, Malgady, & Rogler, 1988), Roberts-2 (Roberts & Gruber, 2007) and the Thematic Apperception Test (TAT; Murray, 1943). The dimensions assessed as well as the specific scoring and interpretation procedures vary by instrument. For the TEMAS and Roberts-2, data are coded on an array of dimensions and aggregated for multiple narratives; data are then compared to norms that measure affect, thinking, social problem solving, and the child's ability to look at a situation, size it up, and provide their impression or solution to the dilemma/problem presented. Data may also be examined for completeness of the story line, consistency of the story with reality, and the qualitative aspects of thinking and affect; these are performance-based characteristics. The TAT is most commonly interpreted qualitatively in clinical practice, although recent work (Teglasi, 2001) has made it possible to provide ratings of the story content according to object relations, emotion, cognition, motivation, and self-regulation. There are numerous subconstructs within each dimension. The ratings are made on a continuum that provides the anchor for comparison among individuals. Although they are not normed, there are empirical data supporting the categories of functioning that guide interpretation (Bassan-Diamond, Teglasi, & Schmitt, 1995; Blankman, Teglasi, & Lawser, 2002; McGrew & Teglasi, 1990; Teglasi & Rothman, 2001).

Other performance-based measures include the Rorschach inkblots and figure drawings. The Rorschach is a perceptual-cognitive task that also elicits projection (Exner, 2003). The information obtained from assessment with the Rorschach is grouped and interpreted in relation to other Rorschach data according to a set of decision rules (Exner, 2003); the data are then interpreted in relation to other information about the child. Although the Rorschach can be used as part of routine assessment practice, it is labor intensive (even with software). For more challenging or difficult clinical problems, it is a useful instrument for school psychologists (Hughes, T.L., Gacono, & Owen, 2007).

Figure drawings have long been part of assessment practice in general, as well as in school psychology practice in particular. A recent review by Flanagan and Motta (2007) identified numerous uses as well as limitations of the data. They concluded that figure drawings are best used in relation with other data as a way to establish rapport and facilitate conversation with the child and to develop hypotheses to be investigated further.

Performance-based measures allow the school psychologist to examine a child's functioning while completing a task.

Assessment of Adaptive Behavior

Adaptive behavior reflects competencies that impact the performance of the activities of daily living that are necessary for personal and social sufficiency (Sparrow, Balla, & Cicchetti, 1984). The components of adaptive behavior follow a developmental trajectory that occurs within a social context; the emphasis is on what the child can do. The assessment of adaptive behavior can be informative in an assortment of clinical situations for intervention planning and is required for the diagnosis of mental retardation. It is evaluated when there are questions about an individual's overall functioning and skills (Sattler, 2002); it is not an area of functioning that is routinely evaluated. While the exact domains assessed vary according to the adaptive behavior scale used, typically considered are daily living skills, communication, cognitive competencies, personal care, interpersonal relations, socialization, health, and safety.

The information is collected by obtaining a report from an important adult, such as a parent, teacher, or other caregiver. Data are obtained either by questionnaire or interview formats. The instruments, such as the Vineland Adaptive Behavior Scales (Sparrow et al., 1984), have acceptable psychometric properties. According to *DSM-IV-TR* (American Psychiatric Association, 2000) a score that is at least two standard deviations below the mean in combination with cognitive or intellectual ability that is also at least two standard deviations below the mean is required to diagnose mental retardation. Important to note is that public schools follow the educational classifications defined by the Individu-

An assessment of adaptive behavior is required to make a diagnosis of mental retardation

als with Disabilities Education Improvement Act (IDEIA, 2004); the criteria used by individual states can differ slightly from the *DSM* criteria.

Assessment of Autism Spectrum Disorders

Autism spectrum disorders are a group of disorders characterized by a person's difficulties in communication, social interaction, and behavioral deficits and excesses. The *DSM-IV-TR* (American Psychiatric Association, 2000) lists five disorders: autism, Asperger's disorder, Rett's disorder, childhood disintegrative disorder, and pervasive developmental disorder, not otherwise specified. The manifestations and severity of these disorders vary, although manifestations typically include behavioral excesses and deficits of notable severity. In recent years detection of these disorders has improved, resulting in a higher incidence of their occurrence than originally thought.

Assessment relies on an array of data and techniques that includes parent interviews, behavior rating scales, a review of medical records, and observation of, and interaction with, the child. Youngsters who are placed on the spectrum are often diagnosed prior to coming in contact with the school psychologist. Because their educational needs are complex, school psychologists have a role in ascertaining their needs and developing treatment plans. These youngsters display a wide array of special needs, with their education taking place in a variety of settings, including public schools.

A full psychoeducational assessment is needed to obtain a functional level as well as a pattern of strengths and deficits. Functional behavioral assessment (e.g., Miller, J. A., et al., 1998) is needed to develop remedial plans. Completion of rating scales such as the Gilliam Autism Rating Scale, second edition (Gilliam, 2006) or the Childhood Autism Rating Scale (Schopler, Reichler, & Renner, 1988) may have a role in diagnosis and progress monitoring.

Neuropsychological Assessment

Neuropsychology entails the study of brain-behavior relationships. Clinical neuropsychology was defined by the members of the Houston Conference on Specialty Education and Training in Clinical Neuropsychology (Hannay et al., 1998) as "the application of assessment and intervention principles based on the scientific study of human behavior across the lifespan as it relates to normal and abnormal functioning of the central nervous system" (p. 161). From this, neuropsychological assessment encompasses the use of assessment techniques such as interview, observation, standardized testing, and informal assessments (Sattler, 2001) to answer questions about and to plan interventions for behavior related to central nervous system functioning. Domains of functioning typically assessed through neuropsychological assessment include cognitive processes such as memory, learning, phonological processing, visual-spatial thinking, attention, executive functions, cognitive fluency, and processing speed; academic achievement; adaptive functioning; and personality. Based on the previous discussion of CHC theory and cognitive assessment, it may be hard to tell the difference between assessment in neuropsychology and school psychology. The primary differences are the emphasis on central nervous system functioning and the disorders of the central nervous system. This distinction may not be one of choice for school psychologists because "traumatic brain injury" and "other health impaired" are categories of disability under special education law. As such, school psychologists have become increasingly interested in adopting many of the techniques of neuropsychological assessment and are increasingly required to learn associated learning-related sequelae of insults to and diseases of the central nervous system.

As a result of neuropsychological assessment techniques being adopted by more and more school psychologists, school psychologists are increasingly seeking additional board certification credentials as neuropsychologists. This role expansion does not come without some controversy, however. Some of the conflict comes from the dual identity of school psychologists working at both the doctoral and subdoctoral level (Tharinger et al., 2008). Neuropsychology practice by licensed, doctoral-level school psychologists who meet the education and training standards set by the Houston Conference and endorsed by the American Academy of Clinical Neuropsychology are likely not controversial. In fact, one might argue, with the extensive training in assessment afforded most school psychologists, that they should be natural candidates for postdoctoral training in neuropsychology. More controversial is when subdoctoral school psychologists who are certified by only a state board of education use the term *neuropsychologist* to describe their capabilities. Academic training at this level tends to include a single course in the biological basis of behavior coupled with assessment knowledge of modern tests of cognitive processes. As such, the use of some neuropsychological techniques for a limited set of problems is appropriate and postdoctoral training is certainly necessary, but use of the title neuropsychologist by such individuals is controversial in professional psychology.

School Neuropsychology

Consistent with the purpose of school psychology, school neuropsychologists use knowledge of brain-behavior relationships to allow individuals to profit from learning experiences. Miller, D.C. (2007) provides compelling evidence that there is an emerging subspecialty in school psychology called school neuropsychology. He characterizes three levels of school psychologists using neuropsychological principles in the school. First are those school psychologists simply interested in neuropsychology in the schools and they tend to attend continuing education workshops or join special interest groups in neuropsychology. Second are those trained in school psychology with an emphasis in neuropsychology. These individuals would likely be trained in a doctoral-level program that offers the time to take extensive coursework and practica experience in neuropsychology. The final level is a bit farther reaching, suggesting that school neuropsychology is a specialty unto itself, distinct from either school psychology or pediatric psychology. Miller, D.C. (2007) points out that because this level is far-reaching, current practices likely fall into only one of the first two categories. Supporting the trend in school neuropsychology has been the publication of several books that cover school neuropsychology, including *School Neuropsychology: A Practitioners' Handbook* (Hale & Fiorello, 2004), *School Neuropsychology Handbook* (D'Amato, Fletcher-Janzen, & Reynolds, 2005), *Essentials of School Neuropsychological Assessment* (Miller, D.C., 2007), and *Best Practices in School Neuropsychology* (Miller, D.C. 2010).

Assessment Techniques in Neuropsychological Assessment

Psychology has seen a burgeoning range of options for standardized, norm-referenced tests that are applicable for neuropsychological assessment. The history of neuropsychology is beyond the scope of this chapter, but tests of cognitive ability such as the Wechsler series have been a part of neuropsychological assessment since at least the 1950s. As previously discussed, modern tests of cognitive ability are based on CHC theory and measure much more isolated cognitive processes, making them valuable to neuropsychological assessment. New tests and test batteries continue to be developed with the goal of reducing the measurement of irrelevant variance to the construct of interest so that individual cognitive processes can be assessed as cleanly as possible. When the demands of a particular test require several cognitive abilities, neuropsychologists rely on task analysis and triangulation with other tests to determine which cognitive ability is accounting for problems in performance (Hale & Fiorello, 2004).

In addition to traditional test batteries of cognitive abilities like the Wechsler, Stanford-Binet, and Woodcock-Johnson, there are now several standardized, norm-referenced test batteries for neuropsychology. These test batteries have taken neuropsychological tests that have been in use for years and updated them and introduced more comprehensive normative groups. This has been a boon for neuropsychologists, but it is necessary to maintain vigilance regarding the reliability and validity of these tests. Table 3.3 lists tests of cognitive processes and brain-behavior relationships typically used by school psychologists.

TABLE 3.3 **Test Batteries of Neuropsychological Functioning Used by School Psychologists**

TEST	COMPOSITE SCORES	AGE RANGE
NEPSY—II	1. Attention and Executive Functioning 2. Language 3. Memory and Learning 4. Sensorimotor 5. Social Perception 6. Visuospatial Processing	3–16 years
Dean-Woodcock Neuropsychological Battery	1. Total Motor Index 2. Impairment Index	4 years–Adult
Tests of Memory and Learning—II	Core Indexes: 1. Verbal Memory Index 2. Nonverbal Memory Index 3. Composite Memory Index Supplementary Indexes: 1. Verbal Delayed Recall 2. Learning, Attention, and Concentration 3. Sequential Memory 4. Free Recall 5. Associative Recall	5–59 years
Wide Range Assessment of Memory and Learning—II	1. Verbal Memory Index 2. Visual Memory Index 3. Attention/Concentration Index 4. Working Memory Index 5. General Memory Index	5–90 years
Delis-Kaplin Executive Function System	9 Independent Subtests	8–89 years

Linking Assessment Data and Intervention

Although psychoeducational evaluations that are conducted to determine eligibility for special education must be comprehensive and multifaceted by law, the main reason assessment data are collected is to use the information to improve the child's or adolescent's functioning. To accomplish this the school psychologist must have considerable knowledge about both assessment and intervention. A solid understanding of what was assessed and what was not assessed is essential. A solid understanding of interventions and what might be accomplished is also essential. Given the wide variety of referral questions and assessment data that school psychologists encounter, this task may be formidable because an equally broad knowledge of assessment and intervention is necessary.

> School psychologists must be proficient in both assessment and intervention to successfully use evaluation data to improve student functioning.

There are several ways in which this might be accomplished. Because there is a potentially wide array of problems identified by assessment data, having several possible means in one's practice repertoire to accomplish the task of linking assessment data to intervention selection is wise. Specific assessment data can be linked to specific interventions in a one-to-one correspondence format, based on research. This is essentially the aptitude-by-treatment approach; and although it has considerable appeal, data supporting it are lacking. Another way would be to identify a number of interventions that are supported by research to address (i.e., remediate or treat) a particular problem that was identified by the assessment data. This premise underlies the Woodcock Interpretation and Instructional Interventions Program (Schrank, Wendling, & Woodcock, 2008), which is software that generates a psychoeducational report and instructional recommendations comprised of well-established empirically supported interventions. Such an approach could be utilized without software. A third means is to develop new assessment materials, standardize them, and subsequently develop interventions that follow directly from the data yielded. This is the basis for the Social Skills Intervention System (SSIS; Elliott & Gresham, 2008). A fourth option is to select particular techniques and/or strategies to address the deficits identified by the assessment data and to use these to develop or build suitable interventions.

Each of these approaches could be utilized to develop Individual Education Programs (IEPs) for special education students, or to provide recommendations to guide parents and teachers for youngsters whose difficulties are less complex than special education needs. In addition, any of these approaches could be utilized to generate suggested recommendations for an out-of-school service provider, such as a tutor or independently practicing psychologist.

Each way of linking assessment and intervention described has benefits and limitations. Aptitude-by-treatment models may have face validity and appeal, despite, as some argue, the lack of systematic data (Reschly, 2008) Interventions may often be selected based on practitioner preference or experience. The linking of empirically supported interventions to test data has science supporting it, but there may be youngsters whose testing profiles do not mesh well with the pool of interventions. Offering an intervention that is specifically linked to test data has scientific support, but it will be appropriate for only selected situations. The last approach, based on clinical judgment, is not systematic, and it can vary across school psychologists. All interventions should be evaluated during implementation via progress monitoring, although this may not occur as frequently as is desirable.

The current trend in schools is to utilize empirically supported interventions in prereferral situations as well as for IEPs. This follows from the Individuals with Disabilities Education Improvement Act (IDEIA; 2004). Schools typically rely upon software to develop IEPs. Based on the child's needs (management, academic, physical, social) and assessment data, overarching goals, short-term objectives, and specific interventions are selected from a menu.

An additional concern is that any circumscribed approach linking assessment and intervention may oversimplify the child's difficulties. For example, a child may have difficulty with math skills but may also have underlying anxiety that requires treatment. Because most psychoeducational evaluations assess a wide variety of constructs, multiple conclusions may be drawn from the same data set, making it possible to offer a broader service that reaches beyond the referral question. Yet some psychologists might argue that using psychoeducational assessment in this manner is an inefficient process because many constructs that may or may not be fully relevant to the referral question are typically assessed. Others might argue that it is wiser to assess an array of constructs in the event that there are secondary areas of concern that need to be identified. Oversimplification can be limited if the school psychologist maintains a broad perspective, considers long- as well as short-term solutions, and weighs competing hypotheses about the child's functioning. Although these are important, the large caseload in school settings and the emphasis on results can mitigate against this approach being the norm rather than the exception.

Strengths and Limitations of Psychoeducational Assessment

As alluded to throughout this chapter, there has been some controversy among school psychologists about the value of psychoeducational assessment versus curriculum-based assessment and functional behavioral assessment. We find all of these forms of assessment to have their place in school psychology. In fact, psychologists such as Smith and Handler (2007) have argued that these forms of assessment should complement each other and can successfully be integrated. That said, much of the criticism of psychoeducational assessment and comprehensive psychological and neuropsychological assessment comes from a behaviorist viewpoint that supports curriculum-based and functional behavioral assessment to the exclusion of other forms of assessment. The primary criticism is that there is a lack of evidence for the linkage between psychoeducational assessment results (usually couched as *g*) and intervention planning. Rather, critics claim that curriculum-based and functional behavioral approaches are much more proximal to the observed problems and define the problem in the context of the immediate learning environment. Applied behavior analysis includes many valuable techniques; however, as the cognitive and biological basis of the behavior revolution (Miller, D. C. , 2007) has shown us, much more is going on than behavioral consequences and there is an enormous literature on the linkage of processing deficits and successful interventions (e.g., Shaywitz, 2003). Thus, consistent with the ecological-transactional model described in chapter 2, a truly comprehensive assessment should include implementation of interventions in the learning environment with progress monitoring, and should these interventions fail despite being implemented with integrity, a comprehensive psychoeducational assessment is warranted. The comprehensive assessment is conducted to determine the factors that account for the refractory nature of the problem and to make recommendations to reduce their impact. Critical to school psychology is that comprehensive assessment be clearly linked to interventions and a treatment plan (e.g., individualized education program) based on the findings of the assessment data.

FOUR

Assessment Strategies II

There are several purposes for this chapter: (1) to define and discuss problem-solving methodology for academic and behavioral problems; (2) to explain these research-driven behavioral methods, their link to intervention, and the implications for case conceptualization and reflective practice; (3) to discuss assessment that meets the demand characteristics of the referral question and the implications for case conceptualization and reflective practice; and (4) to provide information on curriculum-based assessment and functional behavioral assessment, as these types of assessment are applications of the problem-solving model.

The assessment process in school psychology practice is changing. As discussed in the previous chapter, some in the field are challenging the use of psychoeducational assessment. Those same individuals strongly support the use of the response-to-intervention (RTI) paradigm. The overarching concept in RTI has been used for some time in both medicine and in cognitive behavioral psychotherapy. Simply, a hypothesis is put forth about a problem, and an intervention to address it is implemented. If the problem remits, the intervention is considered effective, which in turns means the assessment was on target. The current use, which emphasizes educational applications, is more novel and is the focus of this chapter. For purposes of this discussion, an intervention may be considered a planned modification of the environment that was developed to bring about a specific predetermined change (Tilly & Flugum, 1995). Three broad categories, or tiers, provide an organizing framework under which to consider and discuss problems for which interventions may be developed. Tier 1 refers to a problem that exists because the skill has not been taught, Tier 2 refers to a problem that exists because the child in question needs more time (practice) to learn a skill, and Tier 3 refers to the child who continues to display skill deficits despite instruction and prompting. Individual children who manifest Tier 3 problems may benefit from some level of special education.

Case Conceptualization

Assessment and psychological/psychoeducational testing are not synonymous because standardized testing is one type of assessment. Psychological testing as well as other procedures , such as observa-

Three Categories of Problems for Which Interventions May Be Developed

- Tier 1: Child has not been taught the skill

- Tier 2: Child needs more time to learn the skill

- Tier 3: Child has difficulty learning the skill despite instruction and prompting

tions and interviews, can provide the information that drives the assessment. A strong case conceptualization based on hypotheses about the child and his or her functioning (Christ, 2008) is a precondition for a strong assessment. Because assessment and case conceptualization are interrelated activities and central to problem solving (Batsche, Castillo, Dixon, & Forde, 2008), it is important to remain open to the idea of revising the case conceptualization and gathering additional data as data already obtained are interpreted. Therefore, case conceptualization should help the school psychologist plan the assessment, and in turn, the assessment data should be used to provide a descriptive picture of the child (the ultimate goal). An effective case conceptualization will guide the selection of assessment devices and assist school psychologists in showing the pathways from the problem to be addressed to the plan for intervention. Important to note is that the methodology is applicable to academic as well as behavioral problems (VanDerHeyden & Witt, 2008). Currently popular in school psychology are problem-solving methodologies (e.g., Deno, 1995) to guide this process.

Problem Solving

There are five stages in the problem-solving process (Bergan & Kratochwill, 1990; Upah & Tilly, 2002) (see sidebar), and within each stage there are substages. The exact details and nuances of the problem-solving process will vary according to the demand characteristics of the referral question. While there are discrete stages in problem solving, information learned in later stages often necessitates that earlier stages are revisited so that the conceptualization of the problem can be refined accordingly. Clearly operationalized

Stages of Problem Solving
1. Problem identification
2. Analysis
3. Intervention development
4. Implementation
5. Evaluation

goals are set during the stages prior to implementation so that the intervention can be evaluated for effectiveness and a determination made on whether the child demonstrated improvement.

The quality of the data obtained in the stages prior to implementation of the intervention is critical if it is to be effective in the evaluation of interventions. Batsche et al. (2008) note that data serve three purposes:

1. Data must accurately assess the target behavior/skill

2. Data must inform intervention development

3. The data must be sufficiently sensitive to detect growth

Good quality indicators are composed of problem-solving logic and intervention components (Upah, 2008); these are incorporated within an overall assessment of the intervention plan. These indicators include clear definitions that are supported by multiple data sources, analysis of the problem, intervention development that includes goal setting and a means of measurement, and an evaluative component that measures progress along the way while ensuring treatment integrity and an overall evaluation of progress.

Worth noting is that the problem-solving approach has been used in the cognitive behavioral treatment of adult disorders (e.g., Nezu, Nezu, & Cos, 2007). Case conceptualization involves considering the problem from multiple perspectives to capture its complexity and to gain an understanding of the patient's problems; identify the variables that are functionally related to the problems; and determine treatment goals, targets, and objectives.

PROBLEM IDENTIFICATION

Problem identification includes establishing a behavioral definition of the desired behavior, collecting baseline data of both desirable and undesirable behaviors, and comparing the observed behavior to a standard. This permits the school psychologist to determine whether the child exceeds, meets, or falls below expectations. The target behavior may be a desired level of academic functioning (e.g., knowing the multiplication tables), a behavior related to learning (e.g., attending behavior), task completion (e.g., homework), or interpersonal behaviors (e.g., social skills). The hypothesis that the school psychologist makes as to why a particular behavior is not occurring guides the selection of assessment tools/methods. Some data will be available in school records and is essentially archival or anecdotal; that information provides a point of departure to guide the assessment. School psychologists, however, should be open to including additional data sources during the course of an intervention. Moreover, they should also be open to revising their hypotheses because the hypothesis provides the basis for linking assessment to intervention (e.g., Miller, J. A., et al., 1998). The process of ongoing data collection and hypothesis revision can shed light on how an intervention might be improved, or in the worst case scenario, why it might have failed.

Multiple types and sources of data will be used, typically including multiple informants. Observational data that can be readily quantified are preferred. The use of formal tests is limited, although self-report and behavior rating scales (e.g., Behavior Assessment System for Children-2; Reynolds & Kamphaus, 2004) may be used. Methods that enjoy research support are favored (Kazdin, 2001; Kratochwill, 2005); this is consistent with the trend toward evidence-based practice in professional psychology. The methodology of behavioral assessment (e.g., Hersen & Bellack, 1981) is applicable to both academic and behavioral problems because it focuses on observable dimensions that are operationalized with specificity and can be measured. When observers reach agreement (Kazdin, 2001)—that is, they achieve high rater agreement—this is one aspect of reliability. In establishing rater agreement, there must be an adequate sampling of both desired and undesired behaviors for observers to agree that a behavior was in fact observed. In addition, observations of particular behaviors should include at least three data points, although more are desirable.

However, the required accuracy reaches beyond the notion of rater agreement (Cone, 1978). The size of the disparity between the behavior not desired and the behavior desired provides confirmation (or not) as to whether a problem exists in the first place (despite one being reported). Thus, it is important for the measures to be sufficiently sensitive (Skinner, 1957) and there must be accuracy in recording (Cone, 1981). This information is essential if measureable goals are to be set. It is worth noting that procedures for setting academic skills goals for groups of youngsters or individual youngsters are also available (Shapiro, 2008). The same assessment procedures used to gather information can be used to systematically demonstrate the effectiveness of the intervention.

Additional examples of assessment procedures and sources of data may include interviews with the child, parent(s) and teacher (s); observations of the child (preferably under multiple sets of conditions and in multiple settings); and school records. School systems typically have available a wide array of data on children, and some data will have been specifically collected to track growth. School records may also contain anecdotes and disciplinary information, which provide information on prior difficulties and may identify, or at least suggest, strategies or interventions that have worked, as well as those that did not. These resources can suggest hypotheses that guide the assessment as well as provide data on which to base conclusions. The resources selected are integrated in such a way that data are conceptualized in relation to the science base that forms the basis for contemporary school psychology practice (e.g., American Board of School Psychology, 2007). Important to this assessment strategy is that the school psychologist understand the strengths and limitations of the tools and procedures that are selected for assessment. There is a particular emphasis upon the scientific support for using any given methodology and recognition and consideration of the cautions needed when developing conclusions from the data. For these reasons, assessment procedures are specific to the particular situation and may include psychoeducational as well as social-emotional test data. It is desirable for a theoretical framework to guide this process; an array of legitimate theoretical frameworks is available (e.g., social-cognitive theory) to follow. School psychology as a specialty of professional psychology continues to evolve to recognize the importance of ecological-transactional conceptions of problems and this evolution blends well with the current zeitgeist. These transactions necessitate the consideration of multiple variables and contexts that contribute to the problem and its conceptualization. The discussion of problem analysis that follows is intended to be applicable to the theoretical framework of the reader's choice, although the procedures are most readily aligned with the ecological-transactional approach.

Steps for Integrating Data

1. Note whether findings are particularly salient or significant

2. Identify convergent findings

3. Identify and reconcile divergent findings

4. Determine whether additional data are needed to develop a picture of the child and his or her functioning (Riccio & Rodriguez, 2007)

PROBLEM ANALYSIS

Analysis of the data obtained is the next step. The end result of this analysis reaches far beyond a simple listing of the areas of concern and their documentation, often in the form of some sort of "score." Each piece of data must be interpreted in view of, and in relation to, other data. This is a precondition for developing a synthesized product, which reflects the integration of data, whether it is psychoeducational test data, interview data, or data obtained through observational methods. As discussed in chapter 3, integration of data involves a number of steps (see sidebar).

The level of sophistication reflected in the explanation and integration of data is further reflected in the recommendations made. These recommendations for interventions optimize the child's development. Moreover, the sophistication shown in the selection of assessment devices, methods, and data integration bears a relationship to the training, expertise, and theoretical perspectives of the school psychologist. School psychologists are a heterogeneous group in terms of training, additional credentials, experience, and expertise. It is expected, as a matter of course, that the skills of school psychologists show evidence of the ability to use a variety of assessment tools and methods to produce well-conceptualized pictures of children and their behaviors so that the interventions that are developed and implemented are more likely to produce improvement in their lives. Important considerations for assessment and analysis of data are diversity in all of its forms. Nontreatment variables such as the interpersonal skills and effectiveness of the school psychologist also contribute to the breadth and depth of the assessment and the plan for the intervention. Last, the choice of procedures and the eventual case conceptualization should be consistent with the theoretical foundation that is guiding the particular situation.

Interventions are developed as part of an overall plan of implementation. Included are goal setting, the actual intervention, measurement of behavior, and the manner of determining whether the behavior that is occurring furthers the goal. When behavioral principles direct the problem-solving enterprise from start to finish, the link between assessment and intervention is clear because the hypothesis is confirmed by the data obtained (Batsche et al., 2008). Interventions that follow from a well-conceptualized assessment plan may take a variety of forms. Recently, such interventions have come to be referred to as belonging to Tiers 1, 2, or 3 (Fuchs, 2003). The interventions may be broadly categorized as providing an opportunity to learn new skills, providing additional time and practice to develop the emerging skills, and providing an opportunity for additional instruction for those who are still encountering difficulty learning the skill in the first place (Batsche et al., 2008), respectively. These may include providing services to children and youth individually or in groups, providing assistance to school staff or to families, or by fostering interactions among those involved in the child's care and development (e.g., home-school collaboration).

INTERVENTION DEVELOPMENT

Intervention development follows from the assessment data and analysis in that it addresses the referral question and concerns that are illuminated by

Five Properties of an Effective Replacement Behavior

1. It must be behaviorally described

2. It specifies the current level of the child's performance/functioning

3. It specifies a desired level of performance/functioning

4. It compares the child's functioning to that of peers (as a "normative" frame of reference)

5. The replacement behavior represents a measurable difference from the undesired behavior (Batsche et al., 2008)

the assessment and analysis. When the school psychologist is following a behavioral theoretical orientation, the connection between assessment and intervention is direct and specific to the situation. This approach works well with academic skill deficits (e.g., phonological processing deficits, difficulty learning math facts); behaviors that are overlearned, reinforced, and have become habits (e.g., always watching television before doing homework); and executive functioning deficits (e.g., difficulty with self-regulation). Behavioral interventions often rely upon replacing an undesirable behavior with a desirable one. There are five properties of effective replacement behaviors (see sidebar).

Such a model generally works best for academic problems and clearly observable behavioral missteps. It will be less effective for more complex social-emotional problems that contain internalizing as well as externalizing elements. This is an area that the school psychology literature on response-to-intervention has failed to address adequately. An example, provided in the following section, may prove helpful.

Some problems can appear straightforward, as an intervention that increases a desirable behavior or decreases an undesirable one can address the immediate problem as long as the intervention is in place. However, once the intervention is faded, the original problem resurfaces, suggesting that there is at least one additional concern of significance that prompted the negative behavior in the first place. Consider the child who misbehaves in school. She receives considerable attention for her negative behavior. Because this child seeks attention, the plan to reduce the inappropriate attention sought includes replacing it with social reinforcement for appropriate behavior. Visits to the school psychologist provide the social reinforcement. With the immediate need met, the negative attention seeking has now subsided, so the frequency of visits with the school psychologist is reduced and eventfully eliminated. Once the visits are eliminated, the negative behavior resumes. Why might that be? In our hypothetical example, there was an additional concern. As it turns out, the reason the child misbehaved in the first place was because she was angry over a lack of parental attention. There was no intervention in place to address this anger. Thus, there are situations in which failing to uncover an underlying problem sabotages the success of an intervention aimed at addressing the presenting problem. Moreover, it cannot be assumed that if there are multiple related problems in evidence that treating one will address the others. Generalization of a particular behavior to new settings/situations is difficult to achieve (Kazdin, 2001); it is unreasonable to expect that behaviors related to the presenting problem will simply remit.

IMPLEMENTATION

Well-developed interventions must be carefully implemented to be effective. The intervention must be conducted with fidelity; in other words, its integrity must be maintained. According to Gresham, Gansle, Noell, Cohen, and Rosenblum (1993), integrity is "the degree to which an interventions program is implemented as planned." (p. 254). Too often, an intervention is developed and implemented, yet there is no reliable way to know whether it is carried out as intended. Treatment fidelity is important for a number of reasons (see sidebar).

Moreover, careful implementation is essential to obtain data that will enable a scientific evaluation of the intervention (Noell & Gansle, 2006; Telzrow, 1995). Important to this process are the interpersonal skills of the school psychologist. Effective implementation requires that the stakeholders are informed about and understand the intervention. The interpersonal skills of the school psychologist are then drawn upon to ensure cooperation from all stakeholders; this underscores the need for establishing a positive consultative relationship to make it less likely that there will be resistance to carrying out the intervention as intended (Kratochwill, Elliott, & Stoiber, 2002). Inclusion of stakeholders from the outset builds trust and commitment to the process and the intervention. This is extremely important, as well-meaning adults may make decisions about how to carry out the intervention that may end up negatively impacting its evaluation.

Treatment integrity, or fidelity, may be assessed with questionnaires or checklists developed for the purpose (e.g., Telzrow, McNamara, & Hollinger, 2000). Gresham et al. (1993) suggested these guidelines for evaluating treatment fidelity:

1. Develop operational definitions of the parts of the intervention
2. Use direct observation methods that emphasize frequency counts to measure the (non)occurrence of the desired event

> Importance of Treatment Fidelity
> 1. To ensure that the intervention was carried out as intended
> 2. To be able to replicate the results
> 3. To make evaluation of the intervention meaningful
> 4. To assist in developing the conclusions drawn

3. Obtain multiple estimates of treatment fidelity by session and by overall (non)occurrence of the desired event

4. Supplement the data with a self-report from the individual carrying out the intervention

When trained observers are used, the situation should be arranged so that the adults carrying out the intervention and the child receiving it are unaware of the observer; this will help to avoid the possibility of observer-related biases.

EVALUATION

Prior to evaluating the data, it should be ascertained that the data are indeed usable and of high quality. Thus, some assessment of treatment integrity is a precondition to evaluation. It in fact bears similarity to the considerations one would make about psychological test data as to the validity of the testing situation, which is necessary to appropriately interpret the data. Evaluation may be in a variety of formats, which can be crafted to accommodate the particular situation. Thus, evaluation data may be frequency counts of behaviors, interview data that are self-reports or parent/teacher reports, or questionnaires. Data may also be observational. In some instances, standardized (academic) tests might be appropriate, as are local measures and curriculum-based measures. Also important is that data on academic growth be corrected to partition out the growth that would have occurred if there had been no intervention. Those are considerations to be carefully weighed by the individuals who designed the intervention and the those conducting the evaluation. It is possible in school settings that a team approach will be utilized, and that of course requires that all team members have a full understanding of what is to be accomplished and are in agreement as to how it will occur. Last, the data analysis and presentation of the data to stakeholders requires forethought. Among the possibilities is statistical treatment, although graphs and simple pre-post differences may be sufficient to illustrate progress.

Evaluation may be conducted by using the same tools and methodology that were used to gather the data in the first place, and this is in fact preferable (Noell & Gansle, 2006). That scenario lends itself to pre-post evaluation methods and in particular to graphs.

Moreover, it permits each child to serve as his or her own control. Also possible is making use of N = 1 methodology (e.g., Kratochwill, 1977). Each variety of evaluation has its strengths and weaknesses, particularly in regard to validity and replication of results; these can be addressed by school psychologists, and improvements to the intervention can be made. Thus, evaluation of interventions can be part of a cycle of practice allowing ongoing improvements in practice.

The intervention targets carry implications for the evaluations because the type of data collected may influence the choice of evaluation strategy. For example, for academic intervention targets defined as the child meeting or not meeting a criterion, frequency counts and simple differences will work well. If the intervention target is a variable that is expressed in many ways, an evaluation method that is less will likely work better. For example, if the intervention target is a behavior, such as keeping the work area neat, an evaluation method that allows for before and after comparison makes sense. This may take several forms. One would be to create a template for organization that has specific locations for objects; it would then be determined how many objects are placed in the correct spot. It is also possible to take before and after pictures and simply rely on judgment to determine whether progress occurred— and not quantify the progress. The point is that defining evaluations that are meaningful and helpful (important secondary characteristics of evaluation) should be approached flexibly. The following section discusses a specific instance of the problem-solving approach—curriculum-based assessment.

Curriculum-Based Assessment

Curriculum-based assessment (CBA) has been called an informal assessment technique according to Sattler's (2008) pillars of assessment. However, the use of CBA techniques has increased steadily and is a required competency in most school psychology training programs (Hintze, 2009). Curriculum-based assessment has evolved to a highly sophisticated assessment technique with standard stimuli, norms/benchmarks, percentiles, and in some cases standard scores (cf. AIMSweb.com). Further, the data from CBA are used in progress monitoring to determine an individual's response to a particular intervention. Failure to respond to interventions is used in some states as the criterion for qualification for federal special education services. Thus, CBA has come a long way from being an informal assessment technique. This section first describes the typical assessment methodology of CBA. Then, the distinction between specific subskill mastery and general outcomes measurement is discussed. Finally, current national curriculum-based measurement (CBM) databases such as DIBELS and AIMSweb are covered.

TYPES OF CURRICULUM-BASED ASSESSMENT

Curriculum-based assessment is an umbrella term for a set of procedures used to assess student performance in the local curriculum and make instructional decisions based on those findings. A frequently cited definition of CBA is "direct observation and recording of a student's performance in the local curriculum as a basis for gathering information to make instructional decisions" (Deno, 1987, p. 41). The general notion of CBA is to repeatedly assess what is being taught in the learning environment and to make changes to instruction based on those data. There are a number of approaches to CBA, but the procedure is generally the following. First, the academic behaviors and instructional objectives to be assessed are identified. Sometimes the academic behaviors and objectives can be very circumscribed, such as an individual lesson, or they can be more general, such as first grade word reading. Either way, the instructional objects tend to be sequential (Hintze, 2009). Second, probes are developed from the materials actually used in the classroom or curriculum. Probes are brief snippets of the curriculum materials such as passages from a basal reader, spelling words, or math problems. Probes can be made from curriculum material the student has already mastered, the current material being covered in school, and upcoming curriculum material. Third, the learner is asked to read, spell, or compute the problems in a probe for a short period of time, usually one minute. From the probes, accuracy and fluency can be determined. Performance is then categorized into descriptions based on accuracy and speed such as "frustrational," "instructional," and "independent." There are different schemes for categorizing performance, but one example is 80% to 90% accuracy is frustrational, 93% to 97% is instructional, and 100% is independent (Gilbertson, Duhon, Witt, & Dufrene, 2008). Based on these categories it is possible to identify where in the curriculum an individual is performing at each level because the probes are sequenced from the less challenging to more challenging. Applying the principles of zone of proximal development (Wertsch, 1985) and scaffolding (Wood, Bruner, & Ross, 1976), the teacher can introduce new material in the frustrational level and phase out curriculum materials on which the student is independent. Through this continuous cycle the student is motivated to maintain optimal, consistent forward progress through the curriculum.

As noted previously, CBA is an umbrella term that subsumes a variety of curriculum-linked assessment techniques described using different names such as Curriculum-Based Assessment for Instructional Design (CBA-ID; Hintze, 2009). Different forms of CBA can be distinguished on the dimension of scope of instructional curriculum covered—that is, specific subskill versus general outcomes measurement. In an effort to clarify their approach to CBA as a general outcomes approach, Fuchs and Deno (1991) made the case that CBA is focused on short-term instructional objectives or subskills and that curriculum-based *measurement* (CBM), their approach, is focused on more general outcomes to measure long-term goals. Hintze (2009) provides comprehensive coverage of the various approaches to short-term CBA and the method described in the previous section of this chapter provides the typical approach. General outcomes CBA (also called CBM), on the other hand, was designed to respond to concerns about the reliability and validity of CBA as well as the inability for it to answer questions about a teacher's teaching performance writ large (Fuchs & Deno, 1991). To solve these problems, CBM was required to include "prescriptive procedures and long-range consistency" (Fuchs & Deno, 1991, p. 489). Thus, CBM utilizes standardized probes that cover the full range of skills of a particular curriculum. Curriculum-based measurement is now frequently conducted in schools and its spread has been facilitated by the introduction of Internet-based services for conducting large-scale CBM.

LARGE-SCALE CURRICULUM-BASED MEASUREMENT

As described previously, curriculum-based measurement uses standardized probes and covers a range of an academic curriculum. Designing such probes for each classroom or school would be time-consuming and the reliability and validity of probes would likely be compromised. In response, Dynamic Indicators of Basic Early Literacy Skills (DIBELS; Kaminski & Good, 1996) was developed to provide a reliable and valid method to identify children not making adequate progress on learning and that could be used to measure the effectiveness of interventions on basic reading. The system is available on the Internet (https://dibels.uoregon.edu/) and is in wide use. DIBELS is limited to basic reading and provides indicators of phonological awareness, alphabetic principle, fluency with connected text, vocabulary, and comprehension (Kaminski, Cummings, Powell-Smith, & Good, 2008).

Another, more comprehensive, CBM battery is AIMSweb (http://www.aimsweb.com/) which covers reading, spelling, mathematics, and written expression. AIMSweb is also a data management system that allows school districts to monitor all of their students, generate reports, and conduct progress monitoring. The product has been endorsed by the National Center on Response to Intervention as reliable, valid, and suitable for response-to-intervention implementation.

School Psychologists and Curriculum-Based Assessment

It was stated previously that CBA was included in the curriculum of most school psychology training programs. However, curriculum-based assessment tends to be conducted by teachers in general and special education classes. In most school districts early screening for reading problems is conducted when a child enters kindergarten, again by a teacher. Thus, unlike standardized tests of cognitive abilities and achievement, it is unlikely that a school psychologist will be directly administering CBA probes. So what is the role of the school psychologist in relation to CBA? The school psychologist has several important roles regarding CBA, making it critical that they are trained in the psychometric qualities and uses of CBA (A. J. Schmitt, personal communication, July 2009). First, school psychologists work with school intervention teams to interpret CBA data as well as the progress monitoring of data on interventions. Second, they are involved in interpreting the use of CBA in a response-to-intervention model of placing individuals in special education. Third, school psychologists are involved in formative evaluation (Kaminski et al., 2008) in a school district when CBA data are aggregated across classrooms or schools. Each of these is described in more detail in the following.

SCHOOL INTERVENTION TEAMS

School intervention teams, sometimes called prereferral teams, student assistance teams, or response-to-intervention teams, routinely include a school psychologist as a member. The school psychologist lends guidance to the interpretation of CBA data on individuals shown not to be making progress in a curriculum. The school psychologist can evaluate the technical quality of the CBA probes being used, provide consultative advice about effective interventions for the problem, and objectively examine the treatment integrity of interventions. This is a particularly important role when the child is refractory to typical interventions in the classroom. The school psychologist is knowledgeable about the development of reading, math, and writing skills as well as the cognitive processes that underlie these skills. Using this knowledge, the school psychologist helps gauge scaffolding—the support provided at a particular difficulty to help move the learner to the next level of difficulty—and works to ensure that the sequence of learning is developmentally appropriate. The addition of data from a classroom observation by the school psychologist may provide the intervention team with important, objective, contextual information to interpret the problems in poor responses to intervention.

SPECIAL EDUCATION CLASSIFICATION

The 2004 revision of IDEA included the option to use failure to respond to intervention as a criterion for qualifying for special education entitlement. Curriculum-based assessment is commonly used to determine if an individual has failed to respond to intervention. The determination of whether an individual has failed to respond using CBA is done through the use of benchmark goals and aimlines. *Benchmark goals* are the minimum performance within a subskill that a student must achieve to progress in the development of an academic skill (Kaminski et al., 2008). Students functioning below benchmarks need intervention to get back on track. The determination that a student's rate of improvement is adequate to reach a benchmark goal is done visually using a graph with an *aimline*. The graph has time on the x-axis and performance on the y-axis (e.g., words read correctly per minute). Baseline performance is marked by giving the child CBA probes. From this baseline a line is drawn to the goal level of performance at some point in the future. Over time, the student is reassessed using probes to determine whether progress is at least equal to the aimline, suggesting expected progress is being made toward the goal. The integrity of this system should be examined with the help of a school psychologist due to the psychologist's knowledge of development and single-subject research design. Further, the school psychologist will objectively examine the integrity of intervention implementation and progress monitoring processes. If the student appears not to be responding to intervention, modifications to the intervention should be recommended and tried. If the scores on CBA probes persistently are below the aimline it may be determined the student has not responded to the intervention. Thus, once it appears that the more intensive services of special education are indicated, the school psychologist gathers all of the CBA data and progress monitoring to be included in a comprehensive evaluation to make the final determination of qualification for special education services and provide recommendations to the special education team.

FORMATIVE EVALUATION

Individual student data from CBM systems such as DIBELS and AIM-Sweb can be aggregated across a classroom, school, or even district, to evaluate the quality of interventions and instructional support within the system. This process is described by Kaminski and colleagues (2008) as *formative evaluation*. School psychologists have a variety of roles in the process of formative evaluation with CBM. First, the school psychologist provides consultation to the school district on the psychometric proper-ties of the selected CBM procedure to ensure that it will be amenable to aggregation. Second, the interpretation of graphic and quantitative sum-maries of the formative evaluation data should be conducted by individ-uals with expertise in nomothetic research and statistical analysis, such as school psychologists. Finally, the school psychologist may advise policy makers within the district on best approaches to invoking system change with regard to instructional support, interventions, and disability classifi-cation processes.

Functional Behavioral Assessment

Just as CBA is an assessment approach focused on student performance within the local curriculum, *functional behavioral assessment (FBA)* is an assessment approach focused on interpersonal and learning behavior in the context of the local learning environment. As discussed in chapter 2, one of the theories that undergird school psychology practice is learning theory. Functional behavioral assessment is a subset of behavioral learn-ing theory. In general, behaviorism posits that learning occurs as a conse-quence of the interaction of the events in the environment and the behavior. Functional behavioral assessment comes from the behavioral traditions of applied behavioral analysis and functional analysis (Gresham, Watson, & Skinner, 2001). Applied behavioral analysis is a technique in which system-atic observations of behavior are taken under experimental conditions for the purpose of improving socially relevant behavior (Silva, 1993). Func-tional analysis is concerned with both the situation-specific reasons for a target behavior and the relationship between these determinants and the behavior. Thus, functional behavioral assessment is a process of system-atically gathering observations of a set of target behaviors, examining the relationships between these observations and potential determinants, and, based on these relationships, generating hypotheses about the important, controllable, causal functions of the behaviors for treatment planning and progress monitoring (Miller, J.A., & Leffard, 2007).

The Process of Functional Behavioral Assessment

Once a target problem behavior has been identified, the process of FBA pro-ceeds as follows. First, behavioral observations are gathered through direct observation, behavior rating scales, and structured interviews. Each technique provides a means to systematically collect quantitative and qualitative data.

Second, there is a consideration of the potential causes (functions) of the target behaviors and how those causes relate to the target behavior. Data about these potential determinants are gathered through the assessment procedures listed above. Next, integration and interpretation using clinical judgment is employed to make some conclusions about the nature of functions of the target behavior. Finally, behavioral assessment provides the information necessary to allow the clinician to target the functions of the behavior for treatment and measure the target behaviors to monitor progress.

The typical approach to determining the function of the behavior is to observe the antecedents and consequences associated with the behavior in the local environment. Typical causes of behavior from the behaviorist perspective are to get something such as attention or tangible rewards, to avoid something, and self-stimulation (Gresham et al., 2001). Walker and Sprague (1999) argued that the situation-specific functions of behavior should be extended to include nonsituational risk factors such as family dysfunction, emotional dysregulation, and hostile attitudes toward schooling. Miller, J.A., Tansy, and Hughes (1998) made a similar argument and identified eight classes of functions of behavior: *affect regulation/emotional reactivity*; *cognitive distortion*; positive and negative *reinforcement*; *modeling*; *family issues*; *physiological/constitutional* such as physiological and/or personality characteristics, developmental disabilities, or temperament; *communicate need* including functional communication; and *curriculum/instruction*. Each of these areas can be evaluated through the various assessment techniques (observation, interview, record review, rating scales, etc.) to determine whether any or several are accounting for the target behaviors.

Once the function or functions of the target behavior have been identified, interventions are recommended and implemented. Functional behavioral assessment data collection techniques can then be used to conduct progress monitoring of the intervention. Although FBA was originally mandated for behavior problems, Merrell, Ervin, and Gimpel (2006) recommend FBA techniques for academic problems as well. They suggest that there are often behaviorally related causes for problems in learning such as the work being too difficult or the student not getting enough learning support.

School Psychologists and Functional Behavioral Assessment

School psychologists have an obvious role in conducting FBA as they are typically the professionals who conduct the systematic observations in the learning environment. School psychologists are trained to conduct a variety of behavioral assessment procedures including time sampling, frequency coding, partial and whole interval coding, duration coding, and latency coding (Miller, J.A. & Leffard, 2007). Behavioral observation coding can be conducted informally on a piece of paper; also, there are several published approaches that can improve the reliability of observations such as the Behavior Assessment System for Children, Second Edition, Student Observation System (BASC-2 SOS; Reynolds & Kamphaus, 2004) or the Achenbach System of Empirically Based Assessment (ASEBA; Achenbach & Rescorla, 2001) Direct Observation Form.

On student assistant teams that are interpreting FBAs, the school psychologist has a critical role in interpreting the range of data that were gathered. Applying developmental and psychological theory, the school psychologist helps the team narrow down the potential functions of the problem behavior. The school psychologist works with the team to develop a *behavior intervention plan (BIP)* that is implemented to replace the problem behavior with appropriate behaviors to meet the function and ensure that the problem behavior is not reinforced, and to recommend environmental changes that will ensure that the desired behavior receives reinforcement (Gresham et al., 2001). When more comprehensive functions are considered (e.g., distal, emotional, or physiological), the school psychologist works to put together a BIP that may require much wider ranging services such as, for example, cognitive behavioral therapy, coordination with a primary care physician, or systemic change in the learning institution. Nevertheless, functional behavioral assessment is a core school psychology competency that is employed routinely in the school psychologist's work (Merrell et al., 2006).

PART III

Functional Competency—
Intervention

FIVE

Counseling and Psychotherapy in the School Context

There is increased awareness of the need for expanded psychological services in the schools. Mental health problems of youth are a public health crisis; an organized response is needed (e.g., New Freedom Commission on Mental Health, 2003; U.S. Department of Health and Human Services, 1999). Estimates suggest as much as 20% of the school-aged population experiences moderately serious to serious mental health problems. The consequences are at the human level as well as at the financial level. Among these problems are academic failure, bullying, interpersonal problems, substance abuse, dropping out of school, limited vocational success, problems with physical health, and suicide. Highly trained professional school psychologists who are credentialed for school-based practice as well as independent practice may be among the best prepared to deliver these services (Tharinger et al., 2008) because school psychologists are trained as professional psychologists who have an orientation toward, and understanding of, the school setting and its workings. The purpose of this chapter is to discuss counseling and psychotherapy delivered by school psychologists according to their credentials and practice setting.

Interviewing

THE BASIS FOR COUNSELING AND PSYCHOTHERAPY

Interviewing is a means by which information is obtained to clarify presenting problems in ways that provide usable data to develop recommendations to help the child (or adult). A good interviewer will put the interviewee at ease and create a climate in which the child (or adult) will reveal information

RESPECTFUL

R — religious/spiritual identity

E — economic class background

S — sexual identity

P — psychological maturity

E — ethnic/racial identity

C — chronological/developmental changes

T — trauma/threats to well-being

F — family background and history

U — unique physical characteristics

L — location of residence/language differences

that will assist the school psychologist in developing a plan of action that is helpful. There are considerations underlying the interview process that facilitate the process and increase the likelihood of obtaining needed and useful information. These considerations have been described in detail elsewhere (Cormier & Nurius, 2003; Sattler, 1998) and include nontreatment variables such as the therapeutic alliance, therapist behaviors, the arrangement of furniture in the room, proximity of the seating arrangements, and appropriate etiquette when interviewing clients from diverse backgrounds. Ivey, A. E. and Ivey, M. B. (2008) use the word RESPECTFUL as an acronym to guide the processes of interviewing and counseling (see sidebar); this is one model that is useful in school-based practice because of its coverage of diversity. Interviewing is part of most school psychological evaluations and interventions. The basic components of interviewing should be considered and addressed whether the interview is part of a psychoeducational evaluation or part of a series of counseling or psychotherapy sessions.

Important to interviewing (and working with individuals) is for school psychologists to examine their own values, opinions, and feelings about an array of dimensions. It is also important to consider that different life experiences (e.g., trauma) and different family constellations, among other variables, influence one's worldview and ultimately one's interpretation of and response to interpersonal situations.

What Is Counseling?

The American Counseling Association (1997; available at www.aca.org) defines counseling as "the application of mental health, psychological, or human development principles, through cognitive, affective, behavioral or systematic intervention strategies that address wellness, personal growth, or career development, as well as pathology." This definition of counseling is applicable to school psychology practice.

Counseling is a term far more common to school-based practice than psychotherapy. Counseling in schools is generally not intended to be as intense a service as psychotherapy, nor is it necessarily intended to be long term. Counseling emphasizes giving advice, information, or direction (Corsini, 2000). Most counseling in school-based practice is utilized to address a particular problem or concern. In some instances, what is referred to as counseling is behavior management, because that is the terminology used in educational regulations. When counseling is provided as a longer term service in schools, it is typically assigned to address an ongoing concern that emanates from a chronic problem, illustrated by youngster who throws tantrums because he or she has a developmental disorder. On occasion, ongoing counseling is offered to have an understanding relationship in place should difficulties of greater concern erupt with a student. In this circumstance, it is also common for the youngster to know that the counselor, who is an employee of the school, is available on an "open-door" basis should there be the need. This manner of service delivery enables the school psychologist to monitor youngsters over time.

What Is Psychotherapy?

There are numerous definitions of psychotherapy. One definition indicates that psychotherapy is an interpersonal, *relational* intervention used by trained practitioners to aid individuals in problems of living. This includes increasing well-being and reducing subjective discomfort or distress. The process is one that helps individuals discover why they might think, act, or feel in less than optimal or even unsatisfactory ways (Corsini, 2000). Improved insight into problems and their development is important, but it is not necessarily a final goal. A range of techniques are employed to improve *mental health,* reduce problem behavior, improve affect and thinking, improve social, and academic or vocational functioning, and to improve relationships within a family or a peer group. Psychotherapy is commonly linked to a theoretical or research base (Corsini, 1989, 2000). Important to note is that the difference between counseling and psychotherapy is not particularly clear (Corsini, 2000; Tharinger & Perfect, 2005); there may be more similarities than differences, and some professionals may use the terms interchangeably (Tharinger & Perfect, 2005) and unsystematically (Drewes, 2002). Corsini (2000) likens counselors to teachers and psychotherapists to detectives. This conceptualization of counseling fits well with school-based practice in that the credential that permits school-based practice (in most states) is a teaching certification issued by a state department of education (rather than by a psychology licensing board).

Specifically in the school setting, the differences actually have more to do with the depth and intensity of the service and the mental health of the individual in the first place. In some settings, counseling is often conceived as being for those who do not have diagnosable disorders (but may present a problem that is subclinical and needing attention), while psychotherapy is more often the service provided to those with *DSM-IV-TR* (American Psychiatric Association, 2000) disorders. For these reasons, school psychologists (typically at the doctoral level) who are more highly trained in the assessment and diagnosis of psychopathology as well as those who have been trained to conduct psychotherapy can bring more knowledge and skill to the counseling situation, with the hope of providing a more effective service. Schools, however, prefer the term *counseling* and may not encourage the school psychologist to conduct psychotherapy. Nevertheless, school-based counseling should never be utilized as a substitute for out-of-school psychotherapy when this is indicated.

Psychotherapy occurs in an interview situation, the purpose of which is to create a climate for communication that will facilitate behavioral, cognitive, and/or affective change. The desired changes will be a function of the presenting problem and the theoretical orientation governing the psychotherapy session. Specific approaches appropriate to the goals of therapy are used to foster change. Psychotherapy generally occurs on a weekly basis over a period of time. A combination of the theoretical orientation of the therapist, the complexity of the presenting problem, and the child's motivation to change contribute to the duration of therapy. Also important are environmental variables, which include significant adults at home and school; environmental variables can facilitate or hamper psychotherapy.

Are Counseling and Psychotherapy Really Different?

In summary, counseling is an important practice activity of school psychologists. It is a primary means of intervening with youngsters on an individual basis in the school setting. School-based counseling is typically problem focused and its availability is limited to times when school is in session. In contrast, psychotherapy is more typically provided by school psychologists (who are licensed at the doctoral level) outside the school setting who are working in independent practice, clinic, or hospital settings. Its availability is not limited by the school year. It is difficult to clearly define absolute differences between the

Counseling is typically problem focused and only available at the school when school is in session. Psychotherapy is typically provided outside of the school setting by a doctoral-level school psychologist.

practices of counseling and the practice of psychotherapy. The differences may be more about terminology and custom than service delivery.

Important Ingredients in Counseling and Psychotherapy

NONTREATMENT VARIABLES

There are preconditions that permit the counseling or psychotherapy process to go forward, apart from the theoretical framework under which it is conducted. These nontreatment variables are often crucial to the success or failure of treatment and can contribute to differences in responsiveness to treatment across individuals. Among these are rapport between the child (or adult) and the therapist within a context of therapist behaviors that include respect or unconditional positive regard, empathy or accurate understanding, and genuineness or congruence (Rogers, Gendlin, Kiesler, & Truax, 1967). Also important is interpersonal influence (Strong, 1968), characterized by expertness, attractiveness (e.g., social competence, similarity to self, friendliness, appeal as a person) and trustworthiness of the counselor or therapist. Other important non-treatment variables include verbal and nonverbal behavior, the physical/environmental setting, transference and countertransference, attending and listening, and diversity.

Counselors or therapists who are expert, attractive, and trustworthy derive interpersonal influence from power bases that include legitimate power (the role), expert power (competence), and referent power (social competence/ appeal as a person). Nonverbal behavior on the part of the child as well as the counselor or therapist significantly impacts the therapeutic relationship. Thus nontreatment (Cormier & Nurius, 2003) variables such as proxemics, or environmental space (Hall, 1966); kinesics, or body motion (Knapp & Hall, 1997); paralinguistics, or nonverbal vocal cues (Trager, 1958); time (and its cultural implications); and the client's perception of the environment can influence the receptiveness of the child to the interview, which in turn can influence the information shared and what is ultimately accomplished. The counselor or therapist, in turn, may influence the child in that his or her nonverbal behavior provides cues that either encourage or discourage the child (Cormier & Nurius, 2003). The mutuality of nonverbal behavior cannot be ignored.

Transference and countertransference are nontreatment variables that can occur in school-based practice; they may be prompted by verbal as well as nonverbal behaviors of the counselor or therapist. Transference is classically thought of as the child's reenacting a prior way of relating in a novel situation. More important, however, is how it might be used to help the child.

For example, it is important is to be able to help the child see that the expectations he or she is now making of the counselor or therapist are similar to the unrealistic expectations he or she previously held of others (and the converse, if the expectations are appropriate). Counselors and therapists, in turn, must be cautious about countertransference, as negative behaviors that may surface in sessions may be personally bothersome to the counselors and therapists as well. Thus a task for the counselor or therapist is not to allow any evoked negative feelings to adversely impact the service rendered.

Attending and listening by the counselor or therapist is a nontreatment variable that can convey regard, understanding, and empathy and provides a venue for testing hypotheses about the child. Hypothesis testing is important within the context of interviewing, and is essential (Brammer, Shrostrum, & Abrego, 1989; Cormier & Cormier, 1998) for interviews that are part of an intervention. A hospitable climate permits purposeful information gathering because when the child (or adult) reveals concerns, the individual is given assistance in making sense of his or her thoughts, feelings, and actions.

DIVERSITY

(See chapter 11 for a more detailed discussion.) Some variations in behavior and response to treatment might be a function of culture, individuality, and/or worldview (Ivey & Ivey, 2007) and may be best considered from those vantage points. A precondition for being able to benefit from counseling or psychotherapy is readiness. Readiness for members of diverse populations can differ from what might be typical for the White American populations because diversity is not a unitary construct. It introduces a host of additional considerations that may not be operative for White American youth. These considerations can impact a person's likelihood and willingness to engage in the first place as well as being accepting of the treatment itself. Among these considerations are language, culture, worldview, socialization, conditions of immigration, family circumstances (including socioeconomic status), and the person's view of mental health problems and mental health professionals (Dana, 2007; Fuertes, Alfonso, & Schultz, 2007). Any or all of these variables may play a role at some juncture in counseling or psychotherapy. For these reasons, the concept of cultural intentionality (Ivey & Ivey, 2008), defined as the ability to be flexible and have many possible responses to any issue that may be presented, is a useful guide for practice.

Counseling and Psychotherapy Provide Assessment Data

An expectation for contemporary practitioners is that they evaluate their effectiveness. One way to accomplish this is to gather outcome data. The types of data collected, as well as the frequency and number of data points, will vary as a function of the theoretical orientation followed by the practitioner. We focus on cognitive and behavioral practice in this discussion because that has become the most popular modality in school psychology and it is one the most closely aligned with the ideas discussed.

> School psychologists are expected to evaluate their effectiveness by collecting outcome data.

Regulatory requirements (e.g., IDEIA, 2004) and changes and trends in the nature of school psychological practice (e.g., response-to-intervention) have made it clear that school psychologists are expected to obtain outcome data. Outcome data can take many forms; the main requirements are that the operational definition of the behavior is specific enough that observers can agree that the desired behavior occurred, and that the data can be counted. For example, a case in point is the intervention technique known as *rational emotive behavior therapy* (REBT; Ellis, 1994), which often uses counseling and psychotherapy data as an ongoing assessment. Assessment sessions and intervention sessions are not clearly demarcated, as intervention in REBT ideally starts in the first session. The emphasis is placed on variables that have treatment utility (DiGiuseppe, 1990). DiGiuseppe (1990, 1991) explains that assessment in REBT is *dynamic*, meaning ongoing and capturing changes in the client's thinking. In REBT, the therapist frequently tests hypotheses in order to develop an individualized intervention. The hypothesis-driven impressions can change, subject to new information; some of this information comes in the form of data on the effectiveness of interventions, making assessment and intervention interdependent. Additionally, hypothesis-driven assessment is a collaborative activity between the child and therapist that facilitates rapport and the development of the therapeutic alliance, important in nonvoluntary treatment groups such as children (DiGiuseppe et al., 1995).

REBT views children's problems as the result of emotional disturbance, skill deficits, or both. Moreover, it is common for a child to have emotions secondary to the presenting problem or to be upset about the presence of a problem in the first place. A conceptual model that allows for assessment, intervention, feedback, and evaluation seems appropriate in school psychology practice. Children (or adults) can be provided with suggestions to implement and they can then subsequently report on the outcome. At that point, the intervention either continues as initially conceived or it is refined. This is clearly compatible with the response-to-intervention (RTI) framework as applied to a variety of social and academic problems in a school setting, as a particular advantage is that the school psychologist can monitor the intervention closely. Two pitfalls can be avoided: stopping the intervention too soon, and continuing a flawed intervention unnecessarily.

Common Methods or Types of Individual Counseling and Psychotherapy

How does one select which type of counseling or psychotherapy to use? To some extent, the training and theoretical orientation of the school psychologist will be a determining variable. More important for the overall result, however, is the developmental level of the child (Hughes, T.L., & Theodore, 2009). To determine the appropriate treatment, the psychologist needs to assess the willingness of the child or adolescent to engage in psychological intervention. Remember that unlike adults who voluntarily seek help, the child or adolescent is *brought* to the school psychologist's office (DiGiuseppe et al., 1995), often unwillingly. The following sections describe some of the more common child-adolescent psychotherapies.

Some of the more common treatment types used by school psychologists include:

- Cognitive and behavioral therapies

- Psychodynamic psychotherapy

- Client-centered therapy

- Group therapy (children or parents)

COGNITIVE AND BEHAVIORAL THERAPIES

A wide variety of treatments that fall under the rubric of cognitive and behavioral treatment for youth are available. These vary in scope and intensity, as do the range of difficulties that may be treated with them. More cognitively oriented interventions are based on the notion that what one thinks about an occurrence impacts how one might act or feel (Beck & Emery, 1985; Ellis, 1994). Thus, thoughts and behavior as well as thoughts and affect are in a reciprocal feedback loop. Cognitively focused therapy empowers children and adolescents because they learn coping statements to manage their emotions and plan their behavior. Other cognitively oriented interventions such as means-end thinking (Shure, 1992a, 1992b, 1992c) were created so that children or adolescents can anticipate the consequences of a particular behavior. By being able to anticipate the consequences of their actions, they can make appropriate choices. This method can also help in the management of affect in situations over which the child or adolescent has little control.

Care must be taken to make sure that cognitive-behavioral therapy that is cognitively focused is also developmentally sensitive; a child does not develop the ability to take other perspectives until he or she has attained the formal operations stage (Inhelder & Piaget, 1958). Children at the concrete operational level of cognitive ability (approximately ages 8–11) can understand the coping statements and their rationale, making it possible to engage in the dialogue necessary to explore emotions in cognitive terms (e.g., Bernard & Joyce, 1984. It may be important to teach the youngster how to speak about emotions in ways that facilitate therapy (Di Giuseppe, 1990). An important distinction that sets rational emotive behavior therapy (REBT) apart from other cognitive and behavioral therapies is that REBT aspires to address emotions first and practical problems second (Di Giuseppe & Bernard, 1990). Skill development is also addressed second to emotions. Empirical support is noted through a number of studies reviewed (DiGiuseppe & Bernard, 1990; Ellis & Bernard, 2006) that indicate reductions in anxiety and various problem behaviors through the application of rational emotive principles.

Therapists need to remain alert and prime the conversation as well prompt youngsters to use reasoning skills when indicated. Children at the upper limit of the preoperational level (approximately ages 2–7) do best if they are taught to ask themselves questions when upset, such as "Does this help me?" "Is this good plan?" "Will this help me feel better?" "Will this get me what I want?" "Can I stay out of trouble?" Children must also respond to the questions; thus, by having a conversation with themselves, they can respond to situations in ways that are more effective. Youngsters at the preoperational and concrete operational level also do well with adaptations of Beck's cognitive therapy (Beck & Emery, 1985) that rely upon the therapist to model ways of coping (Knell, 1998). For example, the child can observe the therapist interacting with a stuffed animal that is experiencing anxiety, and by seeing how the stuffed animal copes, the child can incorporate that skill (with practice) into his or her repertoire. A concern is that empirical data for this technique are lacking.

Numerous variations are available on cognitive and behavioral therapies that are cognitively or behaviorally focused (or contain elements of both) and that are empirically supported (e.g., Kendall, Aschenbrand, & Hudson, 2003; Lochman, Barry, & Pardini, 2003; Kazdin & Weisz, 2003); the treatments can be for individuals or groups. A full discussion is beyond the scope of this work, but it is useful to mention the elements common to these treatments and which represent important ingredients in most cognitive and behavioral therapies. Among these are (1) parental involvement in treatment, characterized by frequent updates, and opportunities to discuss the treatment while it is occurring; (2) explanation of the treatment and its rationale to both the parent and the child; (3) an assessment process that bears direct connections to the intervention and can be understood by the clients; (4) goals developed by therapist and client that involve clearly specified tasks for the child (and parents) to carry out; (5) opportunities to practice new skills; (6) opportunities for the child (and the parents) to discuss the treatment and its successes and failures; (7) evaluation of the intervention; (8) refinement of the intervention based on the evaluation; (9) planned termination of treatment; and (10) an understanding that additional treatment may be needed to refresh skills at a later date. Assistance with parenting skills and the management of affect in regard to the child/child's problem may also be indicated.

Examination of these common elements highlights what may be a limitation in conducting cognitive-behavioral treatment in the school setting when available treatment times are limited to times when school is in session. Nevertheless, with adequate planning, many of these elements can be included in an intervention. While there are no data available to quantitatively indicate the exact contribution each element will provide to any given treatment, the list of elements does provide practitioners with things to consider including when they develop or refine interventions. At the other end of the cognitive-behavioral continuum, behaviorally focused therapies include contingency management and token economies. These strategies are more often used to manage specific behaviors and may be included in the behavior intervention plan that follows from functional behavior assessment (see chapter 4 for more information).

PSYCHODYNAMIC PSYCHOTHERAPY

The roots of psychodynamic psychotherapy lie in Freud's psychoanalysis, which provides elaborate and rich theoretical underpinnings. There have been numerous adaptations to the original process, as Freud had followers who agreed, yet refined his concepts, while others disagreed. Important is that most of those whose work can be traced back to Freud's' conceptualizations rely on the notion of developing a (possibly deep) understanding of the problem as an important component of treatment. Tension within the individual's personality structure generates stress. Individuals seek pleasure and avoid pain; at times, those goals can be at odds. If pain is broadly conceptualized to include things children do not want to do or are unhappy about, the application of these concepts to a wide array of children's situations becomes apparent.

The process of treatment relies upon a commitment to self-change through self-examination. Treatment must be developmentally appropriate, as young children do not possess the necessary cognitive skills for self-examination.

Moreover, considerable time may be needed to complete the process. These are some reasons this type of therapy will not be a treatment of choice in school settings; the children who need this sort of help the most are also the children who can least afford to be missing instruction in order to receive treatment. It is important to consider that commitment to self-change is necessary; many children do not agree that there is a problem in the first place! This, however, does not preclude the use of the array of personality theories to explain the child's functioning.

CLIENT-CENTERED THERAPY

A central premise of client-centered (or person centered) therapy is that the therapeutic relationship is characterized by empathy, genuineness, and non-judgmental caring (Raskin & Rogers, 1989). This occurs within a context of trust. This trust means that individuals can reach their potential, set their own goals, and monitor their progress. Children are seen as capable of engaging in this model that leads to self-actualization. The counselor or therapist must be congruent in his or her thoughts and behaviors and show the client unconditional positive regard, which is most commonly expressed through empathy. Concepts from client-centered therapy are most commonly applied to children through play therapy (Schaeffer, 1993). Many types of play therapy are available to accommodate the different theoretical orientations of school psychologists and are appropriate for youngsters of different ages; also, an array of specific techniques (Hall, Kaduson, & Schaeffer, 2006) might be employed.

Although play therapy is a common modality for preschoolers and early elementary aged children, youngsters with limited language skills of any age may be candidates for developmentally based variations of play therapy. There is direction available for psychologists who may wish to employ play therapy with youngsters who evidence concerns that are difficult to address directly, such as abuse (Gallo-Lopez, 2000). All employ play as the medium for providing a secure environment to help children express affect and grow (Schaeffer, 1993), to learn about themselves, or to help themselves change (Knell, 1998), often in a specific domain.

In a nondirective model of play therapy, the child directs the course of the session and decides on the activities that will take place in the therapy room. That means that the agenda for a session will be set by the child. A good bit of patience may be necessary on the part of the therapist (and the child's teacher and parents); thus, this is not the model of choice for a referral problem that requires immediate attention. It is more suitable for issues of an enduring nature. Within a climate of unconditional positive regard, the child has permission to say or do anything in the session and not be rejected by the therapist. The underlying trust must first be developed for the child to be willing to take that risk in the first place. The therapist's role is to reflect (i.e., interpret) what the child says in a manner that helps the child come to understand the meaning of what he or she says and does. Play is the medium through which this occurs.

Client- or person-centered treatment might be used with adolescents, particularly those who resist or are reluctant to participate in counseling or therapy. Those who are resistant because their referral concern is acting-out behavior may be more responsive to an approach that provides an atmosphere that is nonjudgmental. Those who are anxious or ill-at-ease may appreciate not feeling pressured and may be more responsive to an approach that is at their own pace.

GROUP THERAPY

Groups are a welcome modality in schools and sometimes the preferred modality (at least from the viewpoint of school administrators) because it is seen as efficient. Groups may be seen as similar to the classroom experience by some; opportunities to role-play and practice skills are facilitated. To facilitate an effective group, school psychologists need to have skills in several areas (Perusse, Goodnough, & Lee, 2009): (1) knowledge of the interrelationship between developmental theory and counseling theories, (2) knowledge about the topic or content of the group, (3) understanding of group dynamics, and (4) understanding the contextual factors that contribute to child and adolescent behavior.

Groups can be developed according to a variety of parameters. The parameters can range from didactic and psychoeducational to psychotherapeutic (Perusse et al., 2009). Possibilities are gender, age, grade, problem, task, and child characteristics, among others. Groups can be used to discuss specific topics (e.g., bereavement) and address skill deficits (e.g., social problem solving, study skills); they can also be used to provide and practice strategies and to encourage children to explore and discuss topics (e.g., disabilities, diversity) of importance. Groups can be organized around affective concerns such as anxiety or anger (e.g., Flanagan, Allen, & Henry, 2010). A group can be time limited (e.g., 10 sessions) or can be open ended. Groups can also be crafted so that members join the group and leave it as appropriate. Groups can be provided for children, teachers, parents, and families, although it is quite common that the scheduling of groups in the school setting coincides with the school day. Thus, groups that involve families and parents who are employed outside of the home are more likely to occur in settings such as independent practice and school-based clinics, which offer services after school hours. The skill and flexibility of the school psychologist leading the group is a key factor to consider when developing it.

When considering implementing a group therapy model, the school psychologist should consider the longevity of the group (purpose of the group, resources needed, when the group will meet) and the criteria for selecting members.

   The longevity of the group is the first item to address. It is important to consider the purpose of the group and the resources needed to sustain it. The time of day that the group meets may impact its longevity, as youngsters who may profit most from groups may also be the same youngsters who cannot afford to miss instruction. Thus a group that takes place during instructional time may be time limited. In contrast, a group that takes place before school, during lunch, or after school is much less likely to be time limited, although the manner in which the end of the school year is addressed should be made clear from the start. In some instances, there are resources to continue running the group over the summer months; important to consider is whether referrals should be made to out-of-school providers for those youngsters needing continued services if the group does not continue over the summer months. The consideration surrounding longevity of the group necessarily impacts who is offered the opportunity to participate in the group in the first place. These issues that surround the longevity of the group would either be managed differently or may not even be applicable in settings that provide year-round services, such as clinics and independent practice.

   Second to longevity of the group, the most important issue is the selection of group members. A screening process that keeps side issues out of the group (e.g., youngsters who are known to get into fights) is preferred, but not essential. Ground rules are needed, particularly around the limits of confidentiality and conduct in the group setting. A useful way to set the rules is to make this one activity for the first session; group members are generally willing to devote time to rule setting, which promotes an important sense of belonging and investment in the group. Rules are also desirable for conduct outside the group; among these is the requirement that members not discuss the workings of the group with third parties. A distinction is necessary in regard to third parties, as it is appropriate for a child to speak about his or her own group experience with his or her parents; however, it is not appropriate to speak about the other youngsters in the group or the information revealed. Thus, it is important to explain and insist upon a culture of "what happens in this room, stays in this room."

The composition of the group may be built around the purpose of the group (Perusse et al., 2009). Youngsters who share similar concerns and interests are more likely to feel comfortable with one another, a good reason for homogeneous groups. Heterogeneous groups can also be effective. If the purpose of the group is to teach a social skill, it may be desirable to have members who function at various levels, because opportunities for modeling are then available. (See the series volume on group psychotherapy for more information.)

GROUPS FOR PARENTS

Parent training is well suited for group intervention. The same parameters that apply to group treatment for youth in regard to selection criteria, ground rules, and so forth are applicable to groups for parents. Groups for parents are often developed around a shared concern, typically related to the difficulties their children are having. The goals of a group for parents can include coping skills, support, empathy, information sharing, and parenting skills. Take care to guard against the group becoming a forum for complaining and venting to the exclusion of substantive goals. Groups to improve parenting skills are common; such groups are useful for parents of children in all age groups—infants and preschoolers to children and adolescents. Particular advantages of groups include the members' opportunities to brainstorm, practice skills, and troubleshoot challenging situations. Moreover, the brainstorming and troubleshooting skills can be learned, and these are important skills that can be useful in new situations that develop at future times.

Parent groups have been successfully used as part of an overall intervention to address childhood difficulties, such as conduct problems (Webster-Stratton & Reid, 2003) and anxiety (Barrett & Short, 2003) Family-based groups are effectively used for the treatment of eating disorders (Robin, 2003) and are a preferred modality for Latino families (Robbins et al., 2003). Family intervention is culturally sensitive, as problems are typically conceptualized as belonging to the family unit rather than the individual child. Common to these groups is a cognitive-behavioral theoretical orientation. Treatment includes explanations and psychoeducation about the presenting problems, and specific skills useful in an array of situations (e.g., reinforcement strategies) are taught, along with the underlying principles and theoretical underpinnings of the skills. Parents/families also learn to work with personal and family strengths, minimize the negative impact of weaknesses, and learn to work together. This overall approach to treatment enjoys empirical support (Kazdin & Weisz, 2003).

EMPIRICALLY SUPPORTED GROUP TREATMENT PROGRAMS

The severity of problems that children and adolescents experience are often on a continuum that ranges from subclinical to clinical. For example, youngsters may have difficulty speaking up in particular situations, while others may have considerable difficulty speaking in many situations. Given that the school setting provides a unique opportunity to reach large numbers of children who present varying levels of similar concerns, group interventions are an appealing option that can span the continuum from prevention to intervention. A number of empirically validated programs are available that consist of lessons that can be used in small groups or large groups such as intact classes (Goldstein 1988; Elliott & Gresham, 2008; Shure, 1992a, 1992b, 1992c; Vernon, 1998). The programs are developmentally appropriate in that versions are offered for different age groups. In addition, the programs generally deal with the development or strengthening of social skills or social problem solving, or the management of negative emotions. An overarching goal of all of these programs is improved interpersonal relations, whether these are with authority figures, such as parents and teachers, or with peers.

Commercially available group treatments that are empirically validated are available (e.g., Elliott & Gresham, 2008; Shure, 1992a, 1992b, 1992c). The treatment packages are composed of an array of specific lessons, complete with instructional materials. Although not common, all of the lessons in these programs can be used; more commonly, particular lessons can be selected or adapted, making the method versatile. The programs are useful across a spectrum of functioning and can be used to strengthen skills and manage emotions in well adjusted youngsters with no apparent clinical concerns to remediating behavioral deficits and excesses for those youngsters who display clinical-level problems.

Some examples of the skills addressed in these programs are as follows. *The Prepare Curriculum* (Goldstein, 1988) addresses developing prosocial skills for reducing aggression, stress, and prejudice. The *Social Skills Intervention System* (Elliott & Gresham, 2008) contains lessons that address cooperation, communication, assertion, responsibility, empathy, engagement, and self-control. *I Can Problem Solve* (Shure, 1992a, 1992b, 1992c) addresses developing alternative solutions, anticipating consequences of behavior, selecting a solution that provides the desired result, and means-end thinking.

The interventions can be conducted by an array of trained individuals that include teachers, school psychology interns, guidance counselors, and so forth. The skill and expertise of the individuals delivering the intervention need to be considered, with training being provided as indicated. Moreover, appropriate supervision and assistance is desirable to maintain treatment integrity, which is important in general, and essential, if the effectiveness of the intervention is to be determined.

Worth noting is that there is an empirically validated treatment program for Latino youth. Cuento therapy (Costantino & Malgady, 2003) is based on using pictorial stimuli that are related to Hispanic folktales; the intervention is delivered by having the participants relate narratives, followed by discussion. As the discussion progresses and takes shape, more effective ways of addressing daily concerns emerge. While developed for Latino youth, there does not appear to be any reason that the methodology could not be used for others groups of youngsters; adaptations in the pictorial stimuli could be indicated.

Counseling and Psychotherapy in the School Context

Schools are community institutions that can provide the setting in which to offer a variety of services to children and adolescents. In some locales, there are school-based clinics that offer physical and mental health services. Even if there is no clinic, counseling and psychotherapy can be incorporated into the life of the school.

Counseling and psychotherapy in the school setting are often time limited. Although these are important to school success and general social-emotional functioning, there are good reasons to deliver it in a time-limited manner. Children and adolescents will likely miss instruction to attend sessions. Although services offered within the school day are convenient, it can be difficult to have parent participation, which research shows is an important ingredient for successful treatment (see Kazdin & Weisz, 2003). School psychologists and school counselors often work under conditions that are prone to frequent interruptions that are not controlled or managed as these might be in clinic settings. Because school professionals, and school psychologists in particular, have competing demands, appointments may not be as regular as they might be in clinic settings. The interruptions can pose additional concerns should the child or adolescent have more complex mental health needs. While confidentiality is kept, it is difficult to arrange things so that others do not see who is frequenting the school offices. Services are not typically available during school vacations. Last, provision must be made to address the mental health needs of the children and adolescents whose presenting problems are not resolved during the school year.

There are positive aspects to school-based services. Services in school settings are quite suited to time-limited approaches. When insurance monies are not involved, there can be considerable flexibility in how services are delivered. Once parental permission is obtained, an open-door policy for services can be made available. Some youngsters can learn to utilize the services on an "as-needed" basis; even young children can learn how to use an office with such policies. This can limit the disruption to the student's instruction. Moreover, these "as needed" appointments can be of durations appropriate to the situation and the age of the child. They also destigmatize the notion of mental health services.

SIX

Interventions

Although assessment is historically and remains an important role for the school psychologist, linking assessment to intervention has been an important advancement in the role over the past 30 years (Power, 2002). Indeed, intervention is a critical component of the problem-solving model of practice described in chapter 4. Over the course of this transition the specialty saw the emergence of *evidence based interventions (EBI)* as a standard. Using the standard of evidence-based interventions, the specialty has seen the development of a vast collection of interventions. School psychologists prescribe the EBIs based on assessment data as well as monitor them via progress monitoring techniques. In this chapter these topics will be discussed followed by descriptions of types of interventions with examples. These types of interventions are classroomwide interventions, family/parent involved interventions, and academic interventions. The chapter concludes with an examination of the role of school psychologists in intervention planning and monitoring, including the research-based evaluation of interventions.

Intervention Defined

Kratochwill and colleagues (2009) stated that intervention refers to "a wide range of prevention, treatment, educational and service programs that are typically used in clinical or educational settings" (p. 497). Thus, interventions may include counseling and psychotherapy, traditional mental health treatments, and individualized or group programs to correct or prevent academic or behavioral problems. As with other health professions, school psychology has worked to identify interventions that meet the highest standards known as evidence-based intervention (EBI; Kratochwill & Stoiber, 2000a; Kratochwill & Stoiber, 2000b). The term *evidence-based intervention* is the most current and recognized term to describe a class of interventions that meets the criteria set by a professional group and has research-based evidence of its effectiveness. For example, Gettinger and Stoiber (2009) identify the following criteria regarding published studies of effectiveness: experimental or quasi-experimental design was used, intervention occurred for a period of time, multiple outcome measures were used, post-intervention and follow-up data were collected, treatment integrity was assessed, appropriate statistical methods were used, the sample size was adequate, and there were significant and meaningful effect sizes of positive change.

Evidence-based interventions are designed to be *effective*. It is important to note the difference between *efficacious* (efficacy/clinical trials or clinical outcomes) and *effective* (effectiveness/clinical utility) at this point (Clarke, 1995). An efficacious intervention has experimental evidence to support it in one or more research studies. This does not necessarily mean it will have the same clinical effect in a nonexperimental setting or in a setting with different participants, that is, in practice. Interventions that have been shown to generalize to different populations in applied settings are described as effective. This distinction is important because the evidence to support an intervention as efficacious may not suggest it will be effective with a particular population with which the school psychologist is working. Referring back to the conceptual framework under which school psychologists work, the ecological-transactional model, each individual and context will likely introduce variables that will have to be considered in the implementation of the intervention.

Because of the many factors that impact effectiveness in practice, Kratochwill and colleagues (2009) point out that a single definition of an intervention is illusive. Consistent with the purpose of school psychology (see chapter 2), Kratochwill and colleagues define a school-based intervention as "the systematic use of a technique, program or practice to improve learning or behavior in specific areas of student need" (p. 502). This definition contrasts slightly with the more general definition previously given, but importantly identifies improvement of learning or behaviors in learning-related settings such as schools. It should also be noted that their definition of a school-based intervention does not include prevention, although prevention of learning or behavior problems in learning-related settings is an essential component of intervention.

Despite the illusiveness of a standard research-based definition for interventions, Kratochwill and colleagues (2009) identify a relatively generic outline for the factors that should be included when defining or implementing an intervention. Specifically, they identify four general factors starting with *inputs*. Inputs include the human, material, and information resources necessary to implement the intervention with integrity. This includes individuals with the time and interest in implementing the intervention, the appropriate materials such as workbooks or videos, and necessary data including previous response to intervention data or other assessment data. The second factor comprises the *components* of the intervention. These include the specific activities of the intervention including teacher, parent, and classroomwide activities. These also may include assessment activities such as progress monitoring. For example, a mathematics intervention may require the student to listen to taped problems and write the answers down on a worksheet as fast as possible while as the teacher charts the student's performance over time (McCallum et al., 2006). Intervention components need to be well operationalized to allow for evaluation of the intervention, to encourage treatment integrity, and to allow for generalization (Kratochwill & Stoiber, 2000a). The next factor is *outputs* and they are divided into short and long-term outputs. Short-term outputs may include progress on incremental subskills or increase proficiency at implementing the intervention by the teacher. Long-term outputs may include the teacher's applying the intervention to small groups of students with similar problems. Finally, there are *outcomes*, which are evidence that the goals of the intervention have been achieved. Outcomes can be very specific to the goal of the intervention, such as "the student completes basic math problems at grade level fluently," or, more generalized such as "the student reaches grade-level performance on all curriculum-related reading expectations."

Factors of Intervention

- Inputs: resources needed to implement the intervention with integrity

- Components: the specific activities of the intervention

- Outputs: short-term and long-term goals of the intervention

- Outcomes: evidence that the goals of the intervention have been achieved

Evidence-Based Interventions

Evidence-based interventions are determined using criteria set by a professional organization that include research-based evidence for the effectiveness of the intervention. The standards by which the research on an intervention is judged to be evidence based has been complicated by a variety of factors such as integrity of the intervention implementation, the settings in which the intervention is implemented, and the severity of the students' problems at the onset of intervention (Hunsley, 2007; Kratochwill & Stoiber, 2000a). These complicating factors make for fertile opportunities for research and to provide the empirical support for an intervention. However, these factors make it difficult to determine whether an intervention has adequate empirical support. Therefore, at this point there is no one set of standard criteria for empirically based interventions. However, there are some guidelines that have been used within school psychology that can guide school psychologists in intervention selection.

When selecting an intervention, choose one that

- Is supported by multiple studies
- Was researched by individuals with similar training and resources
- Is viewed as appropriate and reasonable for the particular problem

MULTIPLE STUDIES SUPPORTING THE INTERVENTION

Interventions that have been supported in studies that take place in various settings and with different populations provide greater support for the potential effectiveness of an intervention in a practical setting. When several research teams verify the intervention, confidence for its effectiveness increases beyond that of studies by a single research team, generally the team that created the intervention. Clarke (1995) identifies many of the barriers to having such evidence of both efficacy and effectiveness across multiple settings. These include a lack of funding support, methodological barriers such as implementing randomized control studies in applied settings, and feasibility of the intervention to be replicated in various settings. Thus, bridging the efficacy-effectiveness gap will likely require school psychology practitioners to partner with researchers to a greater extent (Hughes, T. L., et al., in press).

LEVEL OF TRAINING, EFFICIENCY, AND COST

Intervention studies that implement the intervention with similarly trained practitioners and similar resources as will be found in applied settings bode well for the effectiveness of the intervention. There is concern that when an intervention shown to have efficacy is applied in practice, the teachers or paraprofessionals implementing the intervention may not have the same level of training or attention to implementation guidelines as the research team that conducted the study. Obviously, practitioners have numerous competing demands during the school day, as opposed to research teams that have an intervention protocol as a circumscribed activity while in the classroom. For application in practice, interventions that are inefficient for the practitioner or costly in terms of human or material resources may not be implemented with the same integrity as under experimental conditions.

Thus, studies that have increased external validity in terms of training, efficiency, and cost parity with the applied setting will provide support for the intervention's effectiveness.

INTERVENTION ACCEPTABILITY

Similarly, intervention acceptability is a concern for bridging the gap between efficacy and effectiveness studies. Intervention acceptability is the extent to which the practitioners view the intervention to be appropriate and reasonable to implement for a particular problem or population (Kazdin, 1980; Kratochwill & Stoiber, 2000a; Kratochwill & Stoiber, 2000b). Studies that examine the acceptability of an intervention and find the intervention to be favorable to constituents likely point to an intervention that has a greater chance of being implemented with integrity in practice. Chafouleas, Briesch, Riley-Tillman, and McCoach (2009) examined a new scaled designed to measure aspects of treatment acceptability called the Usage Rating Profile-Intervention (URP-I). In examining the factor structure of the instrument, they identified several corollary aspects of acceptability. The URP-I showed three other important characteristics of intervention usage in addition to acceptability: understanding, feasibility, and system support. *Understanding* has to do with whether the practitioner understands and has the skills to implement the intervention. *Feasibility* refers to whether the intervention can actually be implemented in the context of the learning environment with particular regard to time. Finally, *system support* refers to the practitioner's perception that additional support will be needed to implement the intervention with integrity (Chafouleas et al., 2009). Each of these is a critical feature that the practicing school psychologist takes into account in determining whether to recommend an intervention for use in a local context.

Intervention and Prevention Approaches

In the following sections, we discuss different types of intervention and prevention practices. The types of interventions discussed are classroomwide interventions, family/parent involved interventions, and academic interventions. In each section, conceptual, practical, and methodological considerations that school psychologists make are discussed, followed by example empirically based interventions. The number of available interventions is enormous, and new interventions gain empirical support every day. Thus, the

Types of Interventions

• Classroomwide

• Family/parent-involved

• Academic

intent of this section is to provide a sampling of the possibilities as they relate to the role of the school psychologist.

INTERVENTION AND PREVENTION

Before discussing the different types of intervention, it is necessary to clarify the difference between intervention and prevention. The definition of an intervention was discussed earlier, and from that definition it could be argued that a successful intervention prevents future problems that may be worse and facilitates adaptive success. Thus, the line between intervention and prevention is blurred. This is because, traditionally, there are three levels of prevention: primary, secondary, and tertiary (Merrell et al., 2006; Reynolds et al., 1984). Primary prevention is designed for students without a serious learning or behavioral problem. It is a form of prevention "designed to enhance the delivery of effective instruction and improved school climate" (Merrell et al., 2006, p. 158). *Primary* prevention is administered to the whole system of learners whether it is a classroom, school, or school district. *Secondary* prevention is for students at risk of serious learning or behavior problems. Secondary prevention is designed to respond early to signs of emerging problems to prevent more serious problems from developing. Many interventions have been developed for the purpose of secondary prevention. Finally, *tertiary* prevention is implemented for students with serious, refractory learning and behavior problems. The assumption here is that students requiring tertiary prevention services have already not responded to secondary prevention services. At the tertiary level there is typically a comprehensive assessment that informs individualized interventions. These levels of prevention form the bases of the three-tier approach to intervention known as response-to-intervention (RTI) in which primary, secondary, and tertiary are labeled *universal* interventions; *targeted group* interventions; and *intensive, individual* interventions, respectively (Tilly, 2008). Therefore, as we discuss the different types of interventions it should be clear that most of them could be framed as forms of prevention. It is critical that school psychologists have adopted this prevention view of intervention because a major criticism of mental services in general is that they are not proactive enough and are implemented after a problem has progressed to a serious level (Hunsley, 2007). Further, this prevention approach is consistent with

Three Levels of Prevention

1. Primary—for students without a serious learning or behavioral problem

2. Secondary—for students at risk of serious learning or behavior problems

3. Tertiary—for students with serious, refractory learning and behavior problems

the public health movement designed to use public resources to prevent the emergence of health problems rather than to treat preventable problems after the fact.

CLASSROOM INTERVENTIONS

In the context of a classroom, the transaction among the teacher and the student and the curricular plan comprise the critical variables of teaching and learning. When learning and behavior problems emerge, an analysis of these variables (context, teacher characteristics, student characteristics, and curriculum) will often indicate the source of the problem and guide classroom intervention planning. In addition, Gettinger and Stoiber (2009) identify grouping strategies, motivation, self-regulated learning, and schoolwide characteristics as essential to success in the classroom. *Grouping strategies* in the classroom have to do with the way small-group learning via cooperative learning, as opposed to competitive learning, is implemented. Here the focus is on the transactions among learners in the environment and how those transactions are managed by the teacher. *Motivation* has to do with how students are encouraged to move from a state of extrinsic motivation to intrinsic motivation, as well as the ways in which the teacher avoids repressing intrinsic motivation (Elbow, 1998). *Self-regulation* is a metacognitive skill that allows students to set goals, make a plan to meet those goals, monitor their progress, make adjustments to the plan as needed, and determine when the work is complete. Effective teachers encourage self-regulated learning through modeling, by setting goals in the learning environment, and encouraging self-evaluation of learning (Gettinger & Stoiber, 2009).

The teacher has the responsibility for organizing the classroom into a learning environment conducive to learning and appropriate behavior. School psychologists consult with teachers to help them identify aspects of the classroom management that may be breaking down and causing more general problems. Thus, it is useful for school psychologists to have a schema for what makes up an effective classroom. Such a schema can be used as a frame to conduct informal assessment of the classroom and to target specific classroom interventions. Doll, LeClair, and Kurien (2009) identified the important relational and autonomy-promoting characteristics of effective classrooms. These characteristics are summarized in Table 6.1. Relational characteristics are critical to learning because much of classroom learning is cooperative, students learn appropriate social skills for adaptive success through the relations that make in classrooms, and a positive teacher-child bond has been shown to promote learning and

TABLE 6.1 **Doll, LeClair, and Kurien (2009) Characteristics of Effective Classrooms**

RELATIONAL CHARACTERISTICS	AUTONOMY CHARACTERISTICS
Teachers' Relationships with Students	Shared Expectations for Success
Students' Relationships with Each Other	Shared Goals for Learning
Parents' Relationships with Teachers and Students	Behavior Self-Control

prevent behavior problems. The relational characteristics reported by Doll and colleagues are the teachers' relationships with the students, students' relationships with each other, and parents' relationships with teachers and students. Doll and colleagues examined the literature on self-regulated learning and autonomous functioning and noted a set of important autonomy characteristics that should be promoted in the classroom. Specifically, they identified shared expectations for success, shared goals for learning, and behavioral self-control as critical to developing self-regulated learning in the classroom.

The issues discussed about intervention effectiveness, acceptability, and integrity are very relevant to the selection of classroom interventions. Elliott and colleagues (2002) indicate that in addition to these, intervention resistance and empowerment are also necessary considerations for successfully implementing a classroom intervention. Intervention resistance means that the teacher or whoever is to implement the intervention is actively or passively resisting carrying out the necessary steps to make the intervention successful. Resistance can come from a variety of sources such as the intervention not being a good fit with the classroom environment or the intervention being instituted in the classroom without adequate buy-in from the teacher. This latter point raises the issue of collaborative problem solving in consultation and the notion of intervention empowerment. Teachers should be empowered to implement an intervention and overcome barriers in the classroom by being active participants in the selection and modification of interventions for the local environment.

EXAMPLE CLASSROOM INTERVENTIONS

I Can Problem Solve Curriculum (ICPS)   Teaching students the metacognitive skills of problem solving has a developmental impact across the curriculum. Shure (1992a, 1992b, 1992c) developed the *I Can Problem Solve* (ICPS) curriculum to capitalize on many of the features of effective classrooms just discussed. The curriculum uses an interpersonal approach to teach the cognitive task of problem solving, focusing on how to learn rather than what to learn. This approach involves both the relational and autonomy characteristics described by Doll and colleagues (2009). The curriculum was originally developed for 4-year-old children in at-risk settings such as high-poverty environments. The curriculum has since been extended to intermediate grades and for work with families. ICPS has two sections called pre-problem-solving skills and problem-solving skills and has three general activities: classroom lessons, interpersonal interaction in the classroom, and integration across the curriculum. The intervention typically takes 10 to 12 weeks. Shure (1992a, 1992b, 1992c, 2001) provides evidence that the curriculum is successful at reducing undesirable behaviors, such as poor impulse control, poor frustration tolerance, social withdrawal, and poor peer relations, and increasing generalizable problem-solving skills. Although ICPS has good evidence for its effectiveness for problem solving, a recent study compared it to an emotion-based prevention program (EBP; Izard et al., 2008), suggesting the EBP program was better at developing interpersonal and emotional regulation. The convergence of such approaches may show promise for comprehensive classroom intervention in the near future.

Promoting Alternative Thinking Strategies (PATHS)   Greenberg, Kusché, and Mihalic (1998) developed a highly regarded classroom intervention curriculum designed to improve social competence, emotional intelligence, planning skills, and frustration tolerance and to decrease externalized and internalized behavior problems. The curriculum is a developmentally based comprehensive program that can be implemented from kindergarten to fifth grade. The PATHS curriculum is theoretically integrated and includes social cognition, cognitive development, social-learning theory, and attachment theory. These theories are used to form the Affective-Behavioral-Cognitive-Developmental (ABCD) model used in the curriculum with the aim of teaching children to integrate the four developmental tasks. The second defining characteristic is the eco-behavioral systems model, which is consonant with the conceptual framework of school psychology. The eco-behavioral systems model is used to implement behavioral change through system change and integration throughout the system. Extending the curriculum principles throughout the learning environment to parents and related service providers can enhance the generalization of learning. The program has three major units: Readiness and Self-Control, Feelings and Relationships, and Interpersonal Cognitive Problem Solving. There is also a Supplemental Unit that extends the principles learned in the major units. The program has 131 lessons delivered over 5 years. The PATHS curriculum has an impressive evidence base of both randomized experimental and quasi-experimental studies (e.g., Domitrovich, Cortes, & Greenberg, 2007; Kam, Greenberg, & Kusché, 2004; Riggs, Greenberg, Kusché, & Pentz, 2006) and has been endorsed in the *Blueprints for Violence Prevention* (http://www.colorado.edu/cspv/blueprints/) as a model program.

FAMILY/PARENT-INVOLVED INTERVENTIONS

School psychologists play a critical role in helping parents and families become involved in the education process of their children in general and involving them in interventions in particular. Children whose parents are involved in their education earn higher grades, have better attendance, complete more homework, are more motivated students, have higher graduation rates, and are more likely to attend college (Coleman & Churchill, 1997; Darch, Miao, & Shippen, 2004). Despite these positive effects, many schools find it difficult to maintain parental involvement (Vaden-Kiernan & McManus, 2005). School psychologists can play a critical and active role in encouraging parental involvement in education (Braden, M. D., & Miller, 2007).

Parental involvement or parental engagement in education is a dynamic process that involves the interaction of parents and teachers in which

> **Hierarchy of Parent Involvement**
>
> - Parenting — creating a home environment in which learning can occur
> - Communicating — attending parent-teacher conferences
> - Volunteering — volunteering for different roles in the school or classroom
> - Learning at home — assisting student with homework and ensuring completion
> - Decision making — involvement in school decision making such as serving on school committees

parents work to have an impact on their child's education (Barton, Drake, Perez, St. Louis, & George, 2004). Further, parent involvement can be delineated by degree of involvement. Epstein (1995) provided a hierarchy of parent involvement from least to most involved (see sidebar).

Braden, M.D. and Miller (2007) identified three ways school psychologists work to improve parent involvement in schools. First is teaching parents about the benefits, barriers, and ways to become engaged in their child's school. Psychologists do this through in-service training, parent outreach at parent meetings, and helping teachers draft letters to parents soliciting their involvement. Second, through consultee-centered consultation, school psychologists work with teachers to increase their ability to work with parents. Some teachers experience feelings of loss of control and a need to avoid potential conflict that can prevent the teacher from encouraging parent involvement. (Buerkle, Whitehouse, & Christenson, 2009;

Wheeler & Stomfay-Stitz, 2001) That is, some teachers may feel that the classroom is their domain and may be threatened that parent involvement in the classroom may take away their power in terms of the curriculum or relationships with students. Also, teachers have to cope with many styles of interpersonal communication from parents including confrontive or difficult parents in the course of teaching their students. Some teachers not comfortable with difficult parents will avoid encouraging parent involvement altogether. Through consultation, teachers can learn to reframe their feelings of loss of control and increase their skills at coping with conflict. The third is via parent-centered approaches. The role of the school psychologist affords many opportunities to have formal and informal individual meetings with parents. Through these meetings the school psychologist encourages a culture of trust and openness to parental input. Through modeling this behavior in small groups, the psychologist encourages the parent to generalize these skills to parent-teacher conferences, volunteering, and even decision making in school leadership. Buerkle and colleagues (2009) extend this list of the role of school psychologists in encouraging home-school partnerships to include (1) garnering administrative support, (2) advocating partnerships with the larger system, (3) developing a "family-school team" (p. 671), (4) working to improve problem solving on both sides of the partnership, (5) helping with conflict resolution, (6) providing social support to the families, and (7) helping develop teacher skills to communicate and maintain relationships with the family.

To improve parent involvement in the school, the school psychologist can

- Teach parents ways to become engaged in their child's school

- Work with teachers to increase their ability to work with parents

- Hold formal and informal individual meetings with parents

When parents are involved, they can be included in the intervention process at a number of levels. Much like general parent involvement in school as described by Epstein, involvement in intervention can range from relatively minimal involvement to a level described as "parents as partners" in which the parent has a central responsibility for implementing, monitoring, and maintaining an intervention. The following examines evidence-based interventions designed to improve parent competence through parent training and approaches to engage parents as partners.

Parent Management Training   Parent management training (PMT) programs typically are implemented to reduce conduct-related problems and delinquency in youth. PMT programs typically involve small group sessions that are face-to-face, over the phone, or via the Internet. The sessions are short, such as 1 or 2 hours per week, and include direct instruction, role playing, and social support. When the youth attends the sessions with the parents there is an opportunity for the group leader to coach specific parent-child interactions. In a recent meta-analysis of PMT programs for conduct disorder, Dretzke et al. (2009) examined 57 repeatable randomized controlled trials of PMT programs for preventing youth conduct disorder. Of the PMT characteristics examined across studies, the majority of the programs did not include the child and more than half of them included 10 or fewer sessions. Dretzke and colleagues found that PMT was an effective intervention for children with conduct problems, and measures of problem behaviors such as the Child Behavior Checklist (Achenbach & Rescorla, 2001) showed statistically significant reductions in problem behaviors when PMT was used.

Linking the Interests of Families and Teachers (LIFT)   Eddy, Reid, Stoolmiller, and Fetrow (2003) provide an example of an empirically based intervention that includes a strong parent-involvement component. The Linking the Interests of Families (LIFT) program is designed to reduce aggressive behavior and conduct disorder in youth. The program targets students' poor social behaviors and poor parenting to reduce the risk of the student developing delinquency and antisocial behavior. With respect to parents, the program targets "inconsistent and inappropriate discipline and lax supervision" (Eddy, Reid, & Curry, 2002, p. 41).

Eddy and colleagues (2002) describe the LIFT program as having three components: child skills training, a playground behavior management program, and parent management training. The first two components are interventions implemented in the school setting to develop students' skills and reinforce appropriate and adaptive interpersonal behavior during unstructured activities. The final component, parent management training (PMT), is of interest here. Specifically, PMT in the LIFT program includes group training sessions with parents on a weekly basis. The sessions have a prescribed curriculum focused on appropriate discipline problem solving and further parent involvement. The LIFT program has been studied using randomized control group trials. Results from these studies indicate that students were less likely to be arrested or to begin using alcohol in middle school than were controls (Eddy et al., 2003). In another study, Stoolmiller, Eddy, and Reid (2000) found that students in the LIFT program showed significant reductions in aggressive behaviors on the playground compared to the control group.

Parents as Partners   Consistent with Epstein's (1995) categorization of parent involvement, one level is for the parent to be involved with helping the child learn at home. This is obviously a relatively high level of involvement in Epstein's scheme. This section aims to show the distinction between programs designed to help parents become competent at child rearing (discussed previously) and involving parents in child-focused interventions (Christenson, 1995). When students' parents are enlisted as partners in the treatment process, the students' generalization of learning from school-based interventions is enhanced and the amount (dose) of intervention is increased by being practiced at home as well as at school. In the literature, such descriptions of parent involvement in the treatment of a child include parent participation, parent tutoring, and home-school partnership. At the most basic level, parents are often asked to engage in interventions with their children by helping with homework, playing games to improve learning or behavior, and responding to home notes from the teacher or school psychologist (Alvord & Grados, 2005; Kelley-Laine, 1998). At the next level, parents may meet with the school psychologist to be taught specific intervention techniques. For example, a parent could be taught to help the child segment phonemes in words with a multisensory approach a la Lindamood-Bell (Sadoski & Willson, 2006). School psychologists can systematically provide the training to parents of children who are requiring intensive intervention so that, as indicated, there is increased generalization and the child has increased opportunities to practice new skills. Specifically, Fishel and Ramirez (2005) examined 24 studies of parental involvement broadly defined and found support for the effect of parent tutoring. Although this was a promising finding, they noted significant concerns about the methodological integrity of parent-involvement studies in general and a need to provide more rigorous evidence to reach the level of evidence-based intervention. Similarly, Cox (2005) found in a review of studies that the most effective home-school partnership interventions involved the two-way exchange of information between the family and the school.

ACADEMIC INTERVENTIONS

The nature of interventions discussed next are secondary and tertiary interventions addressing a problem that is either developing or is considered chronic. These are the interventions that would most likely be prescribed by the school psychologist in association with the child study team or as a result of a special education evaluation. In these cases the school psychologist will have an increased role in monitoring the progress of the intervention and serving as a resource to teachers, behavior specialists, and special education teachers through consultative service delivery.

Targeted group and intensive individual interventions for academic problems are too numerous to describe in a single volume, much less this section of a chapter. Such academic interventions have been developed primarily for basic and applied academic skills such as reading, mathematics, and writing. The majority of research has been on reading skills development (Pressley et al., 2009). However, within each of the two general classes of academic skills (basic and applied) are numerous subskills. For example, reading comprehension is a particularly complicated task that include subskills of sound-, letter-, and word-level processing; working memory; rapid automatic naming; vocabulary; word knowledge; and meaning selection (Pressley et al., 2009). For each of these areas there must be assessment by the school psychologist, and there are specific interventions to remediate each. Thus, it can be seen that the range of interventions would greatly expand once one includes the subskills of basic and applied mathematics and written expression as targets of intervention. In addition to academic skills, there are various academic-related interventions with which school psychologists are familiar. In the latest edition of *Best Practices in School Psychology V* (Thomas, A., & Grimes, 2008), a six-volume compilation, volume 4 is dedicated to best practices in enhancing the development of cognitive and academic skills. In that volume, there is discussion of interventions for academic engagement, homework, study skills, early literacy, communication disorders, and low-incidence handicapping conditions.

Burns, VanDerHeyden, and Boice (2008) note that when an academic intervention is implemented for any of these problems, certain characteristics are necessary for an intervention to be effective. First, the intervention must be correctly targeted. A correctly targeted intervention according to Burns and colleagues is one that is focused on the student, the instruction, or the learning environment that is at the root of the problem; it must also be focused on the right problem. Identifying the right problem could be done through assessment including functional assessment (Merrell et al., 2006). Second, the intervention should include explicit instruction. Simply, do not let the student have to figure out what to do. The intervention should be explained in small, manageable steps with enough direct instruction and detail to maximize the student's chance of learning the task. Burns and colleagues recommend guided practice to help the student correct errors until he or she reaches mastery. Third, the intervention should be scaled to provide an appropriate level of challenge. The intervention should be just within the student's frustrational level and allow for appropriate scaffolding within the student's zone of proximal development. Fourth, the student should be provided with frequent opportunity to respond. Various approaches to drill and practice allow the student to benefit from direct engagement with the task and provide an opportunity to rehearse the new learning. Finally, the student must be provided both formative and summative feedback. The student can be given prompts and cues to help him or her focus on the salient aspects of the intervention stimuli as well as feedback on what the student did well and did not do so well on the tasks associated with the intervention.

The Phono-Graphix (McGuinness, C., McGuinness, & McGuinness, 1996) reading intervention provides an evidence-based example of an intensive academic intervention for word reading. There is substantial empirical support for the effectiveness of the Phono-Graphix program (Denton, Fletcher, Anthony, & Francis, 2006; Endress, Weston, Marchand-Martella, Simmons, & Martella, 2007; Wright & Mullan, 2006). The Phono-Graphix program is delivered either one-to-one or in very small groups of two students. The program is intended for school-aged children from kindergarten to high school. Skills taught through the program are phonemic awareness, sound blending, segmenting, and letter-sound correspondence. The program includes 140 sound pictures of phonemes used in English. The sound pictures are taught to the student via direct instruction. Students progress through four levels including two levels of basic codes, one advanced code level, and finally the multisyllabic words level. Each progressive level encourages the student to combine the sound pictures to make increasingly complex words. The Phono-Graphix is an intensive intervention that includes conducting the practice for 1 or 2 hours per day using 40 lessons over 8 weeks of instruction. The program uses a direct instruction paradigm and student errors are corrected with explicit feedback tied to the program stimuli as suggested by Burns et al. (2008).

PART IV

Other Functional Competencies

SEVEN

Consultation

There are several purposes for this chapter. Consultation as a professional activity is examined. The role of consultation specific to school psychology both outside and within schools is addressed. Current models of consultation are reviewed. Consultee-centered consultation, a more complex and sophisticated conceptualization, is visited because of its connection to the competencies in professional psychology. Moreover, considerations in terms of nontreatment variables, which are not a way in which the school psychology literature has addressed practice, are considered. Additional issues of importance, such as diversity and research and evaluation are also discussed.

Consultation is an important professional activity of school psychologists (Reschly & Wilson, 1995); survey data indicate that 20% to 25% of practice activity involves consultation (Reschly, 2000). Consultation occurs in a variety of forms and is applicable in the full array of settings in which school psychologists are employed, including public schools, agencies, clinics, and independent practice. The setting, its culture, and the population served influence the manner in which consultation occurs. Consultation is an indirect service activity; the school psychologist does not work with the target client (most typically a child) directly. He or she uses theoretical and research-based knowledge about development, learning, diversity, and interventions to change the thinking and behavior of the individual consultee (most typically a teacher) who is raising the concern (e.g., Rosenfield, 1987).

The purpose of consultation is to solve problems. This takes place by strengthening the problem-solving repertoire of the consultee (e.g., Lambert, Hylander, & Sandoval, 2004), as in consultee-centered

> Consultation is an indirect service activity. The consulting school psychologist does not work with the target client directly.

consultation, or by working with the consultee to address a specific problem, as in problem-solving consultation (e.g., Kratochwill et al., 2002). The three types of consultation are mental health, behavioral, and instructional. Lambert (2004) describes mental health consultation as including services that are related to the personality and mental health status of individuals, the promotion of mental health, and the interpersonal aspects of the school setting as a workplace (Caplan, 1970). Behavioral consultation (Bergan, 1977) is the process by which strategies are developed to improve the behavior of a child or groups of children. Instructional consultation focuses on academic and behavioral concerns in school settings (Rosenfield, 2002 a, b), thus striving to develop a better fit between the child and the demands of academic learning. In recent years, a fourth model of consultation, eco-behavioral (e.g., Gutkin, 1993; Gutkin & Curtis, 1999; Zins & Erchul, 2002), has emerged. Eco-behavioral consultation emphasizes the (problem) behavior within context rather than something that simply resides within a child. Training in consultation skills, including practice cases and supervision, is an important part of overall pre-service school psychology training.

This chapter addresses consultation as it relates to the professional and functional competencies (e.g., Barber, Sharpless, Klostermann, & McCarthy, 2007; Kaslow et al., 2007), keeping in mind the manner in which consultation is delivered within professional school psychology. Some activities of consultation have been addressed in other chapters; thus, this chapter emphasizes the elements, process, and evaluation of consultation, with a particular focus on the school setting and how consultation is conceptualized in school psychology practice.

Types of Consultation

- Mental health — promote mental health and the interpersonal aspects of the school setting

- Behavioral — develop strategies to improve the behavior of children

- Instructional — address academic and behavioral concerns in school settings

- Eco-behavioral — use behavioral and eco-behavioral principles

Mental Health Consultation

Caplan (1995) indicates that there are four types of mental health consultation (see sidebar).

Similar to other forms of consultation, mental health consultation is an indirect service, as the consultant does not work with the client but rather works though the consultee, who works with the client. Emotional difficulties that the consultee may have are often ascribed to the client. Rather, the consultee's negative emotions, such as anxiety and depression, are displaced onto the client. This variety of consultation would include communication with other professionals, particularly those outside the schools setting, and possibly parents. Within the school setting, mental health consultation is most typically (not exclusively) conducted with teachers and the principal.

Behavioral Consultation

Behavioral consultation emphasizes a functional approach to assessment and intervention (Kratochwill et. al , 2002). Although the initial emphasis is most typically on problem behavior, behavior consultation may include instructional emphases (Kratochwill et. al. , 2002). The aim of this process is to put an intervention in place that addresses behavioral and cognitive factors as these relate to weaknesses in instructional and social functioning. This is accomplished by using the principles of behavior (e.g., Kazdin, 2001) to guide the assessment of individuals, their behavior and its context, all in the service of developing interventions based on this information. Similar to other varieties of consultation, this is an indirect service based on a collaborative relationship between the consultant and the consultee. This variety of consultation is typically conducted with teachers and parents within the school setting as well as outside it.

Instructional Consultation

Instructional consultation is a process that allows the teacher to improve instructional practices to benefit all students in the classroom (Bergan & Schnaps, 1983). The concept was expanded (Rosenfield, 1987) by including an emphasis on the learner and what can be done to improve learning by making the parameters more specific (Rosenfield, 2002a) and by adding steps to the procedure. This occurs according

Types of Mental Health Consultation

- Client-centered — helps the consultee find the best possible solution for the client
- Program-centered — addresses problems in the administration of mental health programs
- Consultee-centered (case) — helps the consultee handle the case better by addressing problems related to understanding, skill, and objectivity
- Consultee-centered (administrative) — focuses on helping the consultee master problems in planning and directing mental health programs

Process of Behavioral Consultation

1. Develop a relationship with the consultee
2. Identify the problem
3. Analyze the problem
4. Implement a plan for solving the problem
5. Evaluate the plan

Five Steps of Problem Solving in Instructional Consultation

1. Entry and contracting
2. Problem identification and analysis
3. Intervention planning
4. Intervention implementation
5. Resolution/termination

to a three-point (triangulated) model that consists of the student, the task, and the instructional strategies, placing the emphasis on the relationship between the task and the learner's skills and the goodness of fit. The work of consultation is to solve problems to improve the goodness of fit when there is a gap between the task requirements and the skills of the learner. A five-step problem-solving process is called upon to determine how this gap might be addressed (see sidebar).

Documentation of the intervention and its progress is often accomplished by using goal attainment scaling. Goal attainment scaling documents progress according to the achievement of subgoals. This variety of consultation is generally limited to teachers within the school setting.

Eco-Behavioral Consultation

School consultation that takes a preventive approach to problem solving, based on cooperative working relationships between the consultee and the consultant that is guided by behavioral and eco-behavioral principles (Zins & Erchul, 2002), is characterized as eco-behavioral. Ownership of the original idea for characterizing this form of consultation as eco-behavioral is unclear (Zins & Erchul, 2002), although Gutkin (1993) has been a strong contributor. Thus consultation is employed to improve the consultee's skills and keep small problems from becoming larger ones. The improvement in the consultee's skills comes after practice using several similar situations, as the literature suggests that generalization of behavior skills does not occur after one trial (Stokes & Baer, 1977).

Zins and Erchul (2002) have identified elements important to conducting consultation effectively. The preventive aspect of consultation includes problem remediation and attempts to strengthen the consultee's skills as well as alter the environmental variables and setting factors that contribute to the problem. Although the services provided are indirect, direct services, such as counseling or crisis intervention, may also be provided. The consultative relationship is cooperative and equal, with the consultant and consultee sharing responsibility. Nevertheless, the consultant needs to exert interpersonal influence so that the relationship can be directive, while remaining cooperative. The problem-solving process is systematic, orderly, and cyclical; all involved are active participants; there is an array of possibilities to consider. The consultant and consultee should also try to identify and address nontreatment variables that could yield negative results (Zins & Erchul, 2002, p. 638).

Eco-behavioral consultation is versatile and can be used with a wide variety of school personnel and parents; it can be equally useful within the school setting as well as external settings.

Consultation in Nonschool Settings

Although the emphasis of this chapter is on consultation in school settings, it is useful to digress briefly to consider consultation in other settings. School psychologists whose practice includes counseling and psychotherapy also practice consultation. That form of consultation is most typically focused on and driven by the client, and is by definition a direct service.

Depending on the theoretical orientation of the school psychologist, it may or may not contain collaborative elements beyond the stage at which treatment goals are set. This is an important consideration because research on the therapeutic alliance predicts that agreement on goals is needed for the alliance to be strong (Bordin, 1994). Another example of direct services in client-centered consulting would be diagnostic and assessment services; those may take place within a school setting or not. An additional example of client-centered consultation is seeking a first (or second) opinion; that will more typically take place in a nonschool setting, but that is not absolute. The knowledge base and expertise of the consultant must be appropriate to the referral question or concern presented.

This conceptualization of consultation includes communication by the school psychologist (who may or may not be a school employee) with other professionals outside the school, such as physicians, to assist the child and/ or his or her parents by providing better services and minimizing duplication and omission of services; it often includes information exchange. School psychologists can provide information on the effectiveness of medication and can assist with treatment compliance in regard to psychotropic medication, stimulants, and medication for chronic conditions, such as diabetes. These are opportunities to collaborate on the child's care.

Consultation in School Settings

Consultee-centered consultation in school psychological practice is an indirect service that most often, although not exclusively (see Lambert et al., 2004, for a discussion), takes place in schools. The consultant must have an appropriate knowledge base that can be used to frame the conversation and the eventual recommendations. The service must be sought by the consultee.

Consultants must have the expertise to deconstruct the concern presented by the consultee and reframe it according to theoretical models and practice strategies that can be utilized in the school setting. The consultant must not be the administrator who evaluates the consultee and the consultant must not be held accountable for the consultee's work (Caplan, G. 1970). The consultant should have training and knowledge that is different from the professional perspective of the consultee. In keeping with this model, school psychologists are appropriate consultants for teachers because they do not carry responsibility for their supervision. There is no requirement for the psychologist to modify the teacher's behavior; the teacher is free to accept or reject the suggestions and recommendations made because the consulting relationship is collaborative and equal. What is important is the presence of a trusting relationship between the consultant and the consultee; this relationship shares characteristics with the therapeutic alliance and can be fostered (or not) by the same nontreatment variables that are important to counseling and psychotherapy (see chapter 5 for a discussion).

The consultant acknowledges and is mindful of the consultee's expertise. The overall objective is to help the consultee improve his or her problem solving—not only to address the immediate concern but also to build a skill set that might be called upon in the future. It is not the consultant's job to provide therapeutic mental health services to the consultee (Lambert, 2004). Consultee-centered consultation is about process, *not* prescription.

Consultee-Centered Consultation

Consultee-centered consultation is one way to broaden the range of services offered by school psychologists. The overarching objective is to help teachers become more responsive to children and their needs by becoming better problem solvers. Essential to the success of consultation is that the manner in which children are referred by teachers for school psychological services be viewed and approached in a way that is different from what is usually done. Rather than immediately referring the child for a full psychoeducational evaluation (only to learn that the child does not meet criteria for special education services), a review of strategies used by the teacher occurs. This review, which is conducted jointly by the school psychologist and teacher is initially intended to "troubleshoot" the situation, not the teacher's instructional skill or the child's strengths and weaknesses. It is common to find that the teacher is stuck in his or her professional relationship with the child (Brodin, 2004).

It is important that the teacher who is the consultee and the school psychologist who is the consultant agree as to the nature of the problem. This is essential because the consultation process is collegial and not evaluative. The consultee and the consultant share responsibility for clear communication; this typically occurs through the consultee's description of the problem and the questions the consultant asks to clarify the information presented. The stage is then set for joint problem solving, part of which is the consideration of alternatives (Rosenfield, 2004).

Within the context of joint problem solving, a number of possibilities may emerge. It may become clear that the problem was not adequately assessed in the first place. The flaws may be in the way the problem was defined or conceptualized or in the assessment process itself, which may not have been sufficiently precise or systematic from the outset. Having insufficient information about the problem or how it might be most effectively addressed also occurs. It is also possible that the goal or expectations for the child were not well defined or conceptualized, or the goal may be too difficult. The point is that collegial discussion is the preferred way to illuminate the facts that describe the presenting problem. Once the facts about the problem are clarified and agreed upon, the teacher consultee and the consultant school psychologist can begin to collaborate and discuss ways to serve the child better; this discussion is not about who knows more but a recognition that different school-based professionals have different training. Knowledge is shared. Important is that the teacher is the instructional expert and has knowledge about pedagogy. The school psychologist, however, possesses different knowledge about assessment, measurement, principles of learning and behavior, and the systematic evaluation of interventions that the teacher may be unfamiliar with. Thus, the breadth and depth of the school psychologist's knowledge base can be used to enhance understanding of instruction and behaviors related to it, improve or modify a plan already in place, or suggest a different strategy altogether. Collegial discussion is the preferred way for it to become apparent that the school psychologist possesses knowledge about assessment and measurement that can be used in the situation in a positive, helpful, and constructive way.

UNDERLYING CONCEPTS AND PRINCIPLES OF CONSULTEE-CENTERED CONSULTATION

Lambert (2004) suggested that a number of variables (see Table 7.1) impact consultee-centered consultation. These variables are not a focus of the

TABLE 7.1 **Elements of Consultee-Centered Consultation (Lambert, 2004)**

- Consultation as a collaborative problem-solving process
- Influence of the organization, system, or context
- Cognition, motivation, and affect of the consultee
- Clear roles for the consultant and consultee
- Focus on the work problems of the consultee
- Consultee's freedom to accept or reject the consultant's suggestions
- Encourage generating alternative solutions
- Problems considered from multiple perspectives
- Training and supervision of consultants

intervention but could be thought of as nontreatment variables that can exert either a positive or negative influence on the consultation situation, similar to what can occur in psychotherapy.

CONCEPTUAL CHANGE

One of the aims of consultee-centered consultation is to effect change in how the presenting problem is conceptualized by the consultee. Change on the part of the teacher consultee is necessary if she or he is to bring about change for the child client. This is accomplished through the dialogue between the consultee and the consultant, which is the catalyst for change (Babinski, Knotek, & Rogers, 2004). It is important for the consultee to own and retain ownership of the problem and the solution (Brown, Pryzwansky, & Schulte, 1998). As a result of the consultation process, however, there may be conceptual changes in the consultant's thinking that could be evaluated using adequate methods (Sandoval, 2004b). Thus, consultation is a learning process (Sandoval, 2004a) for both parties. Because the consultation process is active, any learning that occurs is also active; hence constructivism is one theory of learning that could provide a framework that informs the consultation process (Cobern, 1993). Important to this active learning process is the development of schemata that are cognitive blueprints learned over time and called upon by the individual to negotiate new situations that present a problem to be addressed. Schemata are also subject to revision; thus, consultation can provide the basis for ongoing learning and professional growth. This revision of schemata may represent a paradigm shift (Kuhn, 1962) that sets the stage for ongoing learning and professional growth that are consistent with competent practice.

NECESSARY INGREDIENTS FOR CONCEPTUAL CHANGE

The consultant must have strong interviewing skills (see chapter 5 for a discussion) for successful consultee-centered consulting. These interview skills require creative, incisive, thought-provoking questioning that prompts the consultee to think differently by seeing alternatives. Thus, a task for the consultant is to complicate the thinking of the consultee (Johannessen, 2004) through interviewing. Moreover, the consultant must reframe or reconceptualize the information that the consultee provides. Eventually, this becomes the responsibility of the consultee; the work of the consultant is to guide the consultee through this process, which is one of working through ambiguities and contradictions on how the components of presenting problem are viewed (Thorn, 2004) as a precondition to developmental change. Several conditions must be in place for the consultant to be able to reframe the presenting problem (Johannessen, 2004). These include

1. Having adequate rapport with the consultee

2. Listening to the consultee

3. Reflecting the consultee's concerns

4. Being able to see multiple perspectives

5. Being able to decipher implicit messages in the consultee's verbalizations,

6. Being able to develop hypotheses about the problem

7. Being able to integrate and reintegrate information so as to reconceptualize or reframe the problem

In an ideal situation, the conversation is such that the consultee begins to see the limitations of his or her approach to solving the problem and is now open to a novel conceptualization. Important to developing a novel conceptualization is agreement on the operational terms used by the consultant and consultee because the role of language and how it is used to communicate is noteworthy (Knotek, 2004). When consultation takes place as a team effort (as is now common in schools), these concerns are magnified because there are more points at which the process could go awry. This may include a realization that the problem is more complex than initially thought. The acceptance of the reframed or reconceptualized statement of the problem by the consultee is the first step in conceptual change. This can be accomplished on an individual or group basis (Babinski et al., 2004); the groups provide a nonevaluative situation in which teachers can discuss student learning and behavior problems constructively and collaboratively. The process (Hylander, 2004a) and dynamics of change are complex, containing numerous steps or elements for the consultee—and pitfalls for the consultant. A full discussion is beyond the scope of this chapter.

The skill set needed by a school psychologist to conduct consultee-centered consultation is a complex one that is effectively is developed over time. Duncan (2004, pp. 88–89) has developed a log that, when filled in, requires the consultant to examine the dynamics of the consultee-consultant interaction regarding an array of variables that describe the communication, behavior, and thinking of both the consultant and the consultee. This provides the consultant with a tool that allows him or her to thoughtfully examine and reflect upon the process. The development and honing of a school psychologist's professional practice skills happens via classroom instruction, progressively challenging supervised practice and its review, and practice in the school setting first as an intern and later as an employee. There is no substitute for the experiential component, as this provides conditions under which professional knowledge and wisdom can grow if the school psychologist functions as a reflective practitioner. It is fair to say that the skills of a beginning school psychologist may be merely adequate, compared to the fine-tuned skills of a seasoned practitioner. As with other practice skills, the university training program provides a solid foundation that provides a basis for ongoing professional growth.

Not all consultation situations end happily. The consultation process may fail for a number of reasons. Although these factors are often attributed to the consultee, some may be applicable to the consultant as well. These factors would supersede the technical expertise of the school psychologist in the "how-to" aspects of the consultation process. They are lack of resources, lack of skill to address the problem, and an incomplete, or lack of, understanding about the case; depending on the situation, these factors could apply to either the school psychologist (consultant) , or the teacher (consultee). For example, competing teaching and practice demands, facing a new challenge with student's needs that required new teaching or practice skills, and over-implyfing the needs of the case. One of the consequences of lack of understanding the case can be the psychologist's failure to realize that the consultee does not genuinely want to participate in consultation. Because consultation is a collaborative process irrespective of the variety of consultation, one way to avoid this unfortunate outcome is to ensure that responsibilities for the process, the interventions agreed upon, and the outcomes are clear from the outset (Guva, 2004); if this is not done, the stage is set for failure. Expectations for the process and all involved should be realistic. In the collaborative process, as both participants realize that new insights may emerge, it is sometimes prudent to agree that a revision of those expectations may be necessary.

Moreover, limited professional objectivity in handling the case can undermine efforts to bring about meaningful and positive change. This limited objectivity on the part of both the teacher (consultee) and school psychologist (consultant) may have its roots in schemata that lead the consultee and/or consultant to nonproductive or even counterproductive solutions, a situation that has been described as theme interference (Caplan & Caplan, 1993). Caplan, Caplan, and Erchul (1995) have noted that this last point is of particular difficulty in school settings. It may occur because of an unfortunate reality of school-based practice: the school psychologist is presumed and expected to be able to handle all cases presented, just as a classroom teacher is expected to successfully teach all children in the assigned classroom. That is an unrealistic expectation and it underscores the need for school-based professionals to have support systems available to help them navigate such situations. Similar to most other interventions, consultee-centered consultation is effective in some situations but ineffective in others.

In sum, consultee-centered consultation is an intervention that is also a preventive service (Lambert, 2004). Considering the consultation as an intervention, when the consultee changes his or her thinking and problem solving, he or she will be better able to help the student whose problem led to the consultation in the first place. Considering the consultation as a preventive service, the changes that occur in the consultee's thinking, conceptualizing, and behavior should allow him or her to use these new methods to visualize and address future problems, with beneficial effects. These changes should help to prevent new problems in the school setting.

The Realities of Consultation in the School Setting

Recent trends in the school psychology literature suggest that consultation most often occurs within a collaborative framework, which may differ somewhat from a consultee-centered framework. Irrespective of the variety of consultation, whether it be behavioral (Sheridan, 2000), instructional (Rosenfield, 2002a), eco-behavioral (Zins & Erchul, 2002), or problem-solving consultation (Kratochwill et al., 2002) in nature, the overarching goal of this collaboration (e.g., Gutkin & Curtis, 1999; Medway, 1979) is to more accurately describe the problems so as to develop a more effective solution. Indeed, the recently revised *Best Practices in School Psychology* (Thomas & Grimes, 2008) includes numerous entries on problem-solving consultative activities.

Problem-solving consultation differs from consultee-centered consultation in several respects:

1. Collaboration is a precondition for problem-solving consultation rather than a possible outcome of the consultee-centered consultation process

2. There is decreased emphasis on the professional work problems of the consultee, as compared to solving the problem in short order

3. There is greater emphasis on product than process, making a prescription a possible outcome of the problem-solving process

4. Conceptual change on the part of the consultee (as well as the consultant) that is essential in consultee-centered consultation is not a necessary outcome of problem-solving consultation

5. Consultee-centered consultation emphasizes better understanding of the child (client) by the consultee; problem-solving consultation emphasizes obtaining resources to assist the child (client)

Duncan (2004) discusses the trend toward problem-solving consultation and away from consultee-centered consultation, noting that contemporary conditions appear to expect shared responsibility (between the teacher consultee and consultant school psychologist for assessment, diagnosis, intervention, and overall outcome. One reason this may occur in schools is that from an administrative point of view, the school psychologist's status is equivalent to that of a teacher. That stance downplays, or possibly even ignores, the uniqueness of the school psychologist's knowledge base and training.

Other Variables That Impact Consultation

DIVERSITY

Multicultural consultation occurs when diversity issues are brought to the front. Ingraham (2004) maintains that there are five elements to consider for a successful consultation when issues of diversity are involved (see sidebar).

Important to consider is the point of entry, the development of culturally relevant interventions, and the evaluation of outcomes; each of these parameters is impacted by cultural experiences and expectations.

REFLECTIVE PRACTICE

Reflective practice is an active activity. Garcia (2004) indicates that there are three key elements in reflective practice (see sidebar).

Five Elements of a Successful Consultation

1. The consultant must have an understanding of his or her culture as well as the culture of the consultee

2. The consultant must have an understanding of the consultee's needs

3. The consultant must consider and address the impact of cultural difference (as opposed to similarity) in the teacher-consultee, child-client, and school psychologist-consultant triad

4. The consultant must consider and address issues of context and power within the consultation situation and society

5. Methods to support consultees in their ability to work with diversity, such as careful framing of the problem, use of multicultural consultation strategies, and reflective practice on the part of the consultant are important.

Clear identification of the problem follows from effective questioning of the consultee by the school psychologist consultant, who will ideally revise the conceptualization of the problem as more information becomes available. In general, increased questioning will reveal that the problem is more complex than initially thought. Framing problems is a complex skill because it requires flexibility in thought, and school psychologists will likely view a problem from a different vantage point than a teacher. The differing viewpoints should be used to enrich the overall conceptualization of the problem; in this

Three Key Elements of Reflective Practice

1. Identifying the problem clearly

2. Framing the problem so that it can be viewed from different professional perspectives

3. Engaging in active inquiry rather than evaluation

way it may be possible to broaden the perspective of the consultant and the consultee while reaching consensus. Active inquiry that occurs throughout the consultation process is an essential ingredient of reflective practice because it permits ongoing examination of the data and the hypotheses drawn from it while providing a basis for ongoing integration of data, revision and refinement of hypotheses, and ongoing reconceptualization of the problem as more information becomes available.

Reflective practice can be promoted in several ways (Garcia, 2004). One way is to use a supervision session as an opportunity to teach via coaching. The supervisor models the school psychologist consultant, who is engaging in active questioning and reconceptualizing as well as reframing the problem in light of the new information. A second method to teach reflective practice is through the analysis of logs that are kept by the consultant. The act of writing allows one to look back on one's work and prompts thinking about it that can show how it might be strengthened.

RESEARCH AND EVALUATION

Research and evaluation are not synonymous, although each is an important effort in furthering the field and service delivery. Research is more concerned with furthering the field. Evaluation may focus on individual clients/interventions. Thus, evaluation efforts can be part of a larger research effort. There are three main research paradigms (Hylander, 2004b) (see sidebar):

Three Types of Research

1. Hypothetico-deductive

2. Interpretive

3. Theory generating

Hypothetico-deductive methodology involves scientific hypothesis testing. Interpretive methodology involves providing descriptions and deeper understanding of the problem. Theory-generating methodology seeks to explain processes and outcomes. The optimal programmatic research effort might include all three paradigms. The current zeitgeist is toward problem-solving consultation rather than consultee-centered consultation, which limits the likelihood of interpretive and theory-generating research (Hylander, 2004b). Hylander suggests that constructivist perspectives may prove helpful in the service of generating theory that might explain the role of nontreatment variables in consultation, such as the therapeutic alliance.

Sandoval (2004b) also urges a broader research and evaluation agenda. While behavioral changes in the consultant and the consultee are important evaluation data, particularly in the behavioral tradition, the conceptual changes made by the consultee and consultant may be even more essential. It is obvious that conceptual change on the part of the consultee is a desired outcome of consultee-centered consultation. Preconditions to conceptual change are changes in consultee attitude and affect. Conceptual change on the part of the consultant is important and can be a vehicle for professional growth, which furthers the field and results in better and more sophisticated services to clients. This can be in consultant efforts that deliver validated interventions to a client via the consultee. Service delivery that improves as a result of provider professional growth is essential to competency.

Consultation provides assessment and evaluation data. One way to view consultation is as a growth process first for the consultee and second for the consultant. Because the process of consultation is a professional journey, the progress on this journey can be documented. Each step of the way provides an ongoing assessment. As assessment moves forward, the progress toward the desired goal for the (child) client can be measured. Thus, similar to cognitive behavioral psychotherapy (e.g., DiGiuseppe, 1991), consultation can be a process of ongoing assessment and evaluation. Such a conceptualization permits the consultant and the consultee to think of the process as ongoing learning that can provide the basis for improved services to children on a real-time basis.

EIGHT

Supervision and Management

There are several purposes for this chapter: (1) to define and then discuss supervision and management; (2) to explain clinical and administrative supervision as these apply in professional psychology, and professional school psychology in particular; (3) to provide information on the supervision of externs, practicum students, and interns; (4) to discuss supervision provided to those meeting licensure requirements; and (5) to discuss and explore how reflective practice is promoted and fostered. As with other professional practice areas, the literature on supervision in school psychology is limited. For this reason, supervision literature developed for different varieties of mental health professionals will be incorporated into the discussion.

Supervision and Management

SUPERVISION

According to the Free Management Library (Authenticity Consulting, retrieved November 21, 2008, from www.managementhelp.org/suprvise/ suprvise.htm), one definition of supervision is "the activity carried out by supervisors to oversee the productivity and progress of employees who report directly to the supervisors." Definitions are at issue in the business world because there are numerous definitions of supervision. Similarly, limited consensus as to a single definition of supervision exists in professional practice. Mead (1990) offers one definition of supervision as "the clinical preparation of novice therapists for the practice of therapy" (p. 5). Hawkins and Shohet (2006) note the importance of supervision being provided to those in training so that children receive improved services and, as a corollary, the supervisor furthers his or her own skills. D. E. McIntosh, and Phelps (2000) reviewed definitions of supervision in school psychology and offer this definition: "Supervision is an interpersonal interaction between two or more individuals for the purpose of sharing knowledge, assessing professional competencies, and providing objective feedback with the terminal goals of developing new competencies, facilitating effective delivery of psychological services, and maintaining professional competencies" (p. 33). This comprehensive definition effectively captures the nuances, complexities, and many guises of supervision in school psychology.

MANAGEMENT

According to the Free Management Library (Authenticity Consulting, retrieved November 21, 2008, from http://www.managementhelp.org/suprvise/suprvise.htm) management "refers to the set of activities, and often the group of people, involved in four general functions, including planning, organizing, leading and coordinating activities." Supervision is an activity of managers; thus, there is overlap between supervision and management. A difference is that supervision has a larger hands-on component than management. There is also limited consensus in the definition of management. Some (Authenticity Consulting, retrieved November 21, 2008) maintain that management also includes leadership skills and a vision for the organization. The vision for the organization would include goals and facilitate guidance for those who carry out the work. This guidance is ideally participative and empowering. There are parallels to professional practice in this model.

Clinical and Administrative Supervision in Professional Psychology

Hawkins and Shohet (2006) reviewed supervision and developed a list of qualities needed to be a good supervisor (see Table 8.1).

These characteristics are applicable to both clinical and administrative supervision roles and context, and address a professional skill set that includes interpersonal skills and adherence to ethical principles. Supervision will be most effective when provided within the context of a relationship that has clear expectations but is sufficiently collegial to enable the supervisees to speak comfortably about their successes and failures. Important in this process is the realization that one task of supervision is to promote the growth of the supervisee within a context of appropriate service delivery, while the supervisor's professional growth continues.

Supervision in professional practice occurs in several ways. Administrative supervision includes being accountable to an administrator in matters

TABLE 8.1 **Qualities of a Good Supervisor**

- Flexibility, which includes being open to an array of theoretical concepts and interventions
- The ability to see multiple perspectives
- The ability to work with diversity, in terms of individuals and cultures
- Being broadly knowledgeable about the field
- The ability to manage his or her anxiety (and other negative emotions) and that of others
- Being a continual learner
- Sensitivity to the work context
- The ability to handle power in a nonoppressive way
- Personal characteristics such as patience, humility, and humor

such as compliance with state and federal guidelines, internal procedures in the school or agency setting, timeliness, and meeting deadlines. An administrative supervisor may or may not have professional practice credentials similar to those of the supervisee. Schools and agencies may have multiple levels of supervision, and the complexity, multiplicity, and uniqueness of these levels is far more complex in schools (Harvey & Struzziero, 2000). In agencies, the lead administrative supervisor is typically the (executive) director. The parallel person in a school setting would be the superintendent. These individuals have other persons who have administrative responsibility to act as their agents in many matters, such as pupil personnel directors, special education administrators, and lead psychologists. Administrative supervisors are the public faces of institutions and are responsible for quality assurance and service integrity in a broad manner (Harvey & Struzziero, 2000; Hawkins & Shohet, 2006).

Clinical supervision includes ensuring the quality of services in ways that differ from the goals of administrative supervision. Clinical supervision focuses on practice/practice techniques; it is more collegial than administrative supervision. Thus, a competent clinical supervisor is able to perform the services that are supervised (Knapp & VandeCreek, 2006). Clinical supervision is an interpersonal learning situation that furthers practice skills for both supervisees and supervisors. The supervisee learning spans from didactic work on specific techniques to learning to think and act as an independent professional. In that regard, clinical supervision is a socialization process that can resemble mentoring. Sometimes clinical supervision refers to colleague consultations regarding practice matters; the topics can range from techniques to legal and ethical matters. Clinical supervision between fully credentialed colleagues is a confidential professional situation and its availability is an essential ingredient for successful professional communities. Those who become supervisors often enter that role with little or no training; experience is limited to that of having once been supervised (Knapp & VandeCreek, 2006). Although that situation is changing, as doctoral programs are including supervision skills in the curriculum, supervision is typically learned by doing. Competent supervisors consider the ethical obligations to the clients and the supervisee, reflect on their own practice, and seek supervision of their supervision as needed.

Clinical supervision in professional psychology typically applies to a senior person discussing cases and offering suggestions to a junior person. The junior person may be a trainee, such as an intern, or may be a newly hired school psychologist. In the former case, the intern is expected to follow the supervisor's direction explicitly, as the internship is still part of graduate education and the supervising school psychologist is functioning as a teacher and is the psychologist of record. This means that the supervisor is legally and ethically responsible for the supervisee's work. In the case of the new professional, the supervision is more collegial, although there is some expectation of compliance with suggestions, particularly if the supervision is part of a program arranged to allow the new professional to meet the supervision requirements needed to sit for the state and national psychology licensure examinations. The individual state and national psychology examinations apply to school psychologists at the doctoral level (and is not required if the individual wishes to remain in school-based practice only). School psychologists who are credentialed at the specialist (certificate) level meet all of their supervision requirements while in the training program and are credentialed by state department of education, not a state psychology licensing board. Thus, clinical supervision is desirable, but not required. Harvey and Struzziero (2000) admit that clinical supervision of such school psychologists does not occur often. This is clearly a paradox and a problem for the field of school psychology.

Clinical and Administrative Supervision in School Psychology

Supervision in professional school psychology refers to both clinical and administrative supervision (Harvey & Struzziero, 2000). Clinical supervision for school psychologists includes mentoring and direction on practice techniques and strategies that are appropriate in any professional setting. Supervision is appropriately provided by another professional school psychologist, although some supervision could reasonably be provided to strengthen counseling skills by those who are so trained. It also includes helping the school

psychologist develop an understanding of the educational enterprise and the profession of education;
this facilitates consultation with teachers and makes
the school psychologist more effective. Although that
information is presented in training programs, this
variety of learning while on the job provides a context for learning about education (which in didactic

Clinical supervision for
school psychologists is
typically provided by
another school psychologist
who mentors and provides
practical guidance.

classes often seems quite removed from school psychology). It extends the
training of the school psychologist to that of a more broadly functioning
professional.

Learning on the job is one way to extend professional development
(Chafouleas, Clonan, & Vanauken, 2002). Professional organizations such
as NASP and APA provide guidance as to the frequency and duration of
supervision. NASP maintains that the supervision must be sufficient to
ensure accountability by the school psychologist for the services he or she
provides. For an intern, supervision should be no less than 2 hours per week.
One supervision hour per week is considered desirable for the first 3 years of
employment. It should be a collaborative, peer-driven process that furthers
the professional school psychologist's development period.

The APA (1981) has more specific and stringent requirements for supervision. The APA maintains that all nondoctoral practitioners should receive
at least 1 hour of supervision per week from a doctoral-level psychologist.
While clearly desirable, this is the exception rather than the norm for school-
based practice. Fishetti and Crespi (1999) reported that 70% of a sample of
school psychologists desired such supervision, yet only 10% actually received
it. More recent survey data (Chafouleas et al., 2002) similarly indicate that 60%
of the school psychologists sampled desire supervision; 33% of those individuals reported that supervision was provided by a supervising school psychologist. The vast majority of the remainder of individuals received supervision
from administrators. There is no regulatory requirement for such doctoral-
level supervision because the certificate issued by a state department of education (at the nondoctoral level) is the necessary and sufficient credential for
practice as a school psychologist. Moreover, many school systems do not have
a doctoral-level psychologist on staff. Even when such individuals are on staff
(more common in the Northeast), time within their workday is not allotted
for supervision, nor is the concept of supervision openly supported by school
administrators.

Administrative supervision, however, differs and includes procedures
and policies for the institution and its employees, transcending professional
practice domains. Within public school settings, individuals who have such

administrative responsibilities are generically credentialed as supervisors by their respective state department of education. School administrators are typically also credentialed as a teacher or are (less commonly) credentialed for providing pupil services (such as school psychology). Thus, the educational expertise of the individuals providing administrative supervision is varied; although less common, in some systems it is a school psychologist. School psychologists, because of the nature of their work and the broad reach of their professional responsibilities, are often accountable to multiple administrative supervisors. This typically includes the school principal and the individual who administers special education/pupil services; this latter person may be a school psychologist by training but is often a special education teacher who also has administrative credentials. There is some variation by locality. However, the individual providing administrative supervision is most commonly the school principal, even if the school psychologist reports to someone whose position is within the central administration of the district (such as the pupil services administrator). In either scenario, that individual providing the administrative supervision is not necessarily a school psychologist. Herein lies some complexity.

Because school psychologists are credentialed for school-based practice by state departments of education with the necessary, sufficient, and required credential for school-based practice, the regulations governing their practice certificates are similar to those that are in force for classroom teachers. Results of a survey indicate that over 75% of the responding school psychologists are evaluated by administrators rather than another school psychologist. Moreover, only 45% of the survey respondents indicated that they were evaluated using a method specifically developed for evaluating a school psychologist (Chafouleas et al., 2002.

In some localities, the school psychologist is in the same bargaining unit and on the same salary schedule as teachers. Thus, within the operation of schools, supervision by someone qualified to supervise teachers becomes legitimate—and in many cases is helpful and not problematic. Problems begin when those not trained as school psychologists cross professional boundaries and challenge test interpretation or indicate that the information in a report is incorrect because it is not consistent with their knowledge and experience with the child and his or her situation.

This limited understanding of psychological tests and psychometrics by education professionals who are not psychologists is expected, although those whose training is limited do not always appear to have that understanding. Complexities increase when a situation arises in the school that results in the school psychologist being in a very difficult position because he or she is bound by the APA (APA, 2002) and NASP (NASP, 2000a) ethics codes; these codes do not always mesh effectively with school procedures and situations. The indications in the APA code that the psychologist will work to resolve differences are helpful, but they can still fall short. Happily, the most recent revision of the code (APA, 2002) has explicitly addressed situations that arise in school-based practice by providing specific standards for practice. This will help limit these difficulties for school psychologists; moreover, the code has specifically named school psychologists as being expected to adhere to the code (Flanagan, Miller, & Jacob, 2005). The complexities of supervising school psychologists are discussed by Fischetti and Crespi (1999).

Development of Supervisees and Supervisors

Stoltenberg and Delworth (1987) indicate that the expectations of supervisors from supervisees can follow a developmental trajectory that corresponds to stages in the supervisee's career. The stages culminate in an integrated model. This integrated model brings together domains of professional functioning, as these relate to structures such as the self, motivation, and awareness across the supervisee's developmental level (Stoltenberg, 1993). Supervisors are often seen as consultants by supervisees, yet the actual role of the supervisor is teacher. The model posits that students and beginning practitioners desire help with specific techniques, mid-career practitioners tend to focus upon theoretical models, and those who are most seasoned are typically interested in learning how to integrate theory and practice; thus the tasks of supervision can proceed through stages. Supervisors should adapt the supervisory process as appropriate for the developmental level of the supervisee. Note that student supervisees are typically evaluated, making the relationship with the supervisor one of a teacher, not a consultant.

Supervisors, similarly, pass through developmental stages (Stoltenberg & Delworth, 1987). The stages correspond to (1) being an eager novice supervisor, (2) realizing that supervision is a complex process, (3) realizing that the way to move forward as a supervisor is to make accurate self-appraisals and strive to improve, and (4) developing the ability to adapt supervision practice to fit with the supervisee in terms of the supervisee's professional development, functioning, and culture and theoretical orientation. Seasoned supervisors need to have technical skills, be able to conceptualize how the supervisee approaches clients, and be able to consider the case from the vantage points of client, supervisee, and supervisor. Supervisors also study the supervision literature to assist them in this task (Mead, 1990). The overall process is a task of ongoing development for both supervisor and supervisee.

More recently, a model of supervision derived from Prochaska and DiClemente's (2003) stages of change model for the psychotherapy process has been posited (Aten, Strain, & Gillespie, 2008). The model is composed of six stages:

1. Precontemplation

2. Contemplation

3. Preparation

4. Action

5. Maintenance

6. Termination

The model provides for change and growth in both the supervisor and supervisee, independent of theoretical orientation. Although this model has six stages, there is room for subgoals, making greater specificity possible in matching supervisory interventions to the needs of the supervisee.

Hawkins and Shohet (2006, p. 127) developed a self-assessment tool for supervisors that considers a variety of dimensions: (1) knowledge, (2) supervision management skills, (3) supervision intervention skills, (4) capacities or qualities, (5) commitment to one's own ongoing development, (6) skill development as a group supervisor, and (7) skill development for senior organizational supervisors. This is a potentially useful tool for gauging supervisor growth and development.

Supervision of Externs, Practicum Students, and Interns

Supervision of individuals in university training programs is an important professional activity. University training programs rely upon the expertise of those in the field to provide hands-on experiences and assist in the professional socialization of new school psychologists. The responsibility is considerable, encompassing practice skills and ethics, and should not be assumed lightly. The supervisor's practice should evidence high ethical standards, following both the American Psychological Association code (APA, 2002) and the code of the National Association of School Psychologists (NASP, 2000b). Compensation and release time for supervision is not necessarily granted by the setting in which the supervisor is employed. Thus, those who volunteer to be supervisors are genuinely interested in working with students and must have excellent time management skills because they still have a primary obligation to their employer to serve children and their families. University training programs may provide honoraria, free courses, or conferences for the supervisors as a way of maintaining a community and providing recognition. Some institutions may appoint them as affiliated faculty.

The university training program has obligations to fulfill both to the student and the supervisor. It is important to recognize that the supervision enterprise involves balancing the needs of multiple stakeholders. There is the obligation to the supervised student to ensure that he or she receives an appropriate training experience that meets the standards of the accrediting bodies and the profession. There is also the obligation to the supervisor that the training program provide a student who has met program standards and will not be a liability to the supervisor. There is the obligation to the children who are served by the student. For these reasons, and others (which are discussed in the chapter on teaching), the placement site must be visited by a representative of the training program and there must be evaluation of the student and the supervisor.

WHO ARE EXTERNS AND PRACTICUM STUDENTS?

Externs and practicum students are those enrolled in doctoral and specialist programs who are gaining hands-on experience in the setting prior to the internship; the terminology differs according to the type of graduate training program. Externs are typically enrolled in doctoral programs, and this is a term that is used across specialties of professional psychology. Specialist programs in school psychology tend to use the term *practicum*; hence practicum students are enrolled in programs that are leading to certification as a school psychologist by a state department of education. (The term *intern* is used at both the specialist and doctoral level; the internship is the culminating practice component of training and is generally a year-long experience.) Externship and practicum often take place in university training clinics; the hands-on aspect of training may be embedded within a course. Externship and practicum typically permit students to continue their experience with the concrete aspects of service delivery while allowing and encouraging them to participate in planning the service to be delivered.

Externship and practicum provide opportunity to develop and practice the discrete skills that were introduced in courses. Students practice testing/assessment, counseling, and consultation skills and receive direction and feedback on these without being placed in the practice setting. Skill development occurs for its own sake, without addressing the contextual variables that typically accompany practice, which often link different practice skills. Cases assigned to students are generally not complex clinical problems (for example, not personality disorders or dual diagnoses) but rather problems that can typically be addressed with a good therapeutic relationship and techniques that can be readily learned. Thus, the externship/practicum typically involves services that are provided in relative isolation. Students do not typically experience delivering multiple services to the same client at this time; the reader should keep in mind that school psychologists practicing in school settings may provide different varieties of services to the same child over a period of time. It is more the norm than the exception because school psychologists can follow a child throughout the child's school career (Vane, 1985).

In contrast, the internship takes place in a public school or a clinic or hospital setting that is delivering a range of school psychological services to youth. At the specialist level, the experience is generally in a public school setting, as that is the most likely site for employment. There is greater variety in experience at the doctoral level, although some part of the training often involves exposure to school-based practice. The supervision activities of supervisors and the skills that are emphasized will likely vary according to setting. Both practicum students and interns are evaluated by the supervising school psychologist at the placement site as well as by a university-based supervisor. The evaluation typically consists of completing a rating form that is uniform for all students from a particular training program; the use of other less structured and formalized methods is not precluded. Students may be provided with the opportunity to evaluate the supervisor as well.

SEQUENCE OF SUPERVISION

The progression in training from the classroom to practicum/externship to internship is such that there is a progression in the skill level and type of service provided; similarly, there is a progressive change in the focus, tasks, and types of supervision rendered. Supervisee development follows a progression of stages that begins with self-focus and progresses to client focus, and from focus on single processes to focus on integrating processes (Hawkins & Shohet, 2006). Training in the understanding and application of professional ethics should be infused throughout supervisory experiences (National Association of School Psychologists, 2000a, 2000b).

This process begins with classroom-based instruction; students are given discrete assignments (e.g., giving a particular test and preparing a report) that are graded by the course instructor. The feedback provided to students combined with classroom discussion would constitute supervision. The focus is on skill development and the teaching of theory; these are pre-practicum experiences.

   Course instructors vary in their training and view of the field, representing a diverse group of school psychologists. Some course instructors are academic school psychologists holding faculty positions who have little or no post-degree experience in the delivery of school psychological services; these individuals may not have any more training than they received in their own university training program, and they did not aspire to be practitioners. These individuals are primarily researchers. That is the least common scenario. More common are those who hold faculty positions and have had experience as practicing school psychologists. The range of experience can be quite varied, as some decide that school-based practice is not a preferred career path, and move on to academia after a few years; those individuals tend to be fairly recent graduates. Others may have extensive experience as practicing school psychologists and have chosen later in their career to work in academia. Still others prefer to continue working in the schools and teach courses as adjunct faculty. All of these individuals have something unique to offer supervisees. The varied emphases in supervision can reflect the theoretical cutting edge information that appears in journals or information that is common practice in schools blended with considerable experience and wisdom gained as a practitioner. In the latter case, the emphasis is more applied. All the various types of experiences are valuable.

   The actual supervision during practicum and internship is most typically 2 hours per week face-to-face with the supervisor. Discussion of cases in terms of administrative and clinical procedures commonly takes place. In regard to administrative procedures, the supervisee learns how to meet specific setting mandates as well as government/regulatory mandates. Clinical supervision addresses the clinical work of case conceptualization, assessment, diagnosis, treatment and its evaluation, and the role and management of nontreatment variables. Attention must be given to the supervisee's feelings about the clients and his or her willingness to accept supervision. Supervisees must also learn appropriate professional boundaries. There is a paucity of literature to guide supervisory practice (Harvey & Struzziero, 2000), although some resources are available (e.g., Haboush, 2003; Harvey & Struzziero, 2000; Ward, 2001).

EXTERNSHIP/PRACTICUM

The supervision provided to externs and practicum students can help them strengthen their ability to develop rapport with clients, increase their effectiveness in selecting data sources, and assist them in integrating the data more effectively to facilitate case conceptualization. The supervision should also include developing professional judgment so that the extern or practicum student begins to anticipate common problems that occur in practice and to start thinking about the case in more than one way so that the plan that was made for assessment, consultation, or intervention can be adapted as appropriate.

The externship or practicum is also important in helping the student make the transition from doing homework to providing a professional service. An important task at this level of professional training is for the supervisor to model research-based practice. Sometimes adaptations are needed for research-based professional practice to be smoothly integrated into an existing setting. Thus, seasoned practitioners do not always use the research in the exact manner intended by those who produced the research. While not optimal, this is not necessarily a problem, providing the supervisor communicates to the supervisee the rationale for the adjustment *and* takes that into account when considering outcomes. An important task in supervision at this level is to show the supervisee that there is more than one way to approach a practice situation and one way is not necessarily better than the others.

INTERNSHIP

Internship is the culminating professional practice opportunity afforded to school psychology students. By the time a student reaches internship, he or she must be able to provide basic school psychological services; the supervisor should not be spending time teaching basic skills, such as psychological testing or interviewing. The supervisor's job is to help the student learn how to provide a range of school psychological services and begin to function independently in the setting. Thus, toward the end of the internship experience, the intern should assume the role of building psychologist (although still under supervision) and become the "go to" person. This latter task is important because once employed in school settings, the novice school psychologist is expected to function independently, and there is no requirement that certified school psychologists be supervised by psychologists. Thus, the internship can become an even more important training experience as it often marks the end of ongoing supervision by an experienced school psychologist.

Skill development during the internship should include experience with the broader functioning of a school so that the new school psychologist at least becomes familiar with the daily workings of a school. Opportunities to provide the full range of school psychological services are important as are opportunities to provide multiple services to individuals. Interns should be able to plan a service and be able to offer a rationale as to why they chose a particular path over others. Interns should gain exposure to a wide range of problems.

Supervision for Those Meeting Licensure Requirements

This type of supervision can take one of two forms: a formal postdoctoral year or supervision by a colleague employed by the setting to provide the face-to-face supervision required by licensing boards. Formal postdoctoral positions are developed to teach the psychologist specialized skills that would not be typically taught in the doctoral training program. For the school psychologist this might include neuropsychological assessment or cognitive behavior therapy. Such positions are typically housed in hospital settings. In the other situation, an individual school psychologist who has a doctorate gains employment in a school or hospital/clinic setting and receives supervision from a colleague in the setting. That colleague may or may not be the administrative supervisor. In this type of supervision, the supervisee typically learns to negotiate the setting and has the opportunity to strengthen his or her practitioner skills. Supervision is face-to-face and takes place for 1 to 2 hours per week. At the conclusion of that year, the supervisor completes paperwork that is submitted with the supervisee's application for licensure as a psychologist.

Fostering and Promoting Reflective Practice

As indicated earlier, supervision should be a learning practice. This applies to both the supervisee and the supervisor. *Reflective practice,* ideally done by all practicing psychologists, involves critiquing practice by ongoing evaluation, the purpose of which is to subsequently refine professional practice. The supervisor can teach the supervisee how to engage in reflective practice in several ways: (1) by encouraging the supervisee to consider and reflect upon what will be the most and least challenging professional tasks while under supervision, (2) through listening to the supervisee and by asking carefully crafted questions of the supervisee when discussing cases, and (3) by modeling how a reflective practitioner functions. Reflective practice also includes helping the supervisor improve by considering supervision through an autocritical lens. Supervisors need to be aware of their own processes, and that includes their feelings about supervision, the case presented, and the supervisee (Hawkins & Shohet, 2006). Negative feelings in any of these domains can exert an untoward influence on the entire process. Fortunately, the skill set needed to be a reflective practicing school psychologist and a reflective school psychology supervisor are similar in both instances, although clearly applied in different ways.

Through careful questioning, the supervisee is encouraged to think about practice. It is important for the supervisor to prompt the supervisee to think about the rationale underlying clinical decision making and practice. When a supervisee learns to think about practice in a broad manner, he or she can develop greater competency in professional school psychology than can be acquired by simply applying to a presented situation practice skills that had been taught in isolation. In fact, that latter scenario would have the school psychologist function more like a technician. Also remember that school psychologists have different needs in terms of the activities of supervision than others working in the school system; this underscores the need to distinguish administrative supervision and clinical supervision (Chafouleas et al., 2002).

When a practitioner emphasizes thinking skills and clinical decision making over the delivery of specific services, he or she develops the habit of reflective practice. Such psychologists are more likely to treat each practice situation as unique, as are the individuals who are the consumers of school psychological services. Thus, their approach to practice is marked by flexibility in thinking that is characterized by their ability to consider multiple perspectives; diversity of students, parents, and teachers; and alternative explanations for what is occurring. The ability to apply critical thinking in order to consider the scientific strengths and weaknesses of multiple theoretical perspectives and research findings is important to reflective practice. Flexibility in thinking and willingness to consider incorporating contemporary thought into practice is very important on two counts: consumers of school psychological services benefit from the latest knowledge, while the field of school psychology practice is advanced. The rationale for the clinical decision making that the school psychologist uses may be driven by accepted theoretical knowledge, principles of behavior, and/or specific research findings. The choice of practice strategy/intervention is ideally one that enjoys empirical support.

NINE

Teaching

There are several purposes for this chapter: (1) to discuss the educational levels at which school psychologists are trained, (2) to discuss the similarities and differences between the levels of training, (3) to discuss the complexities involved in training at two educational levels, and (4) to discuss specific issues in training that promote and develop competency and reflective practice, irrespective of educational attainment.

Levels of Training on School Psychology

Within the field of school psychology, faculty are often referred to as trainers. As is the case with other areas of professional psychology, the task of the faculty is multifaceted and complex. Adding to the complexity is that school psychologists are credentialed for practice at two levels: specialist and doctoral. The subdoctoral specialist training is sometimes embedded in doctoral training, particularly when a university offers both levels of training. Subdoctoral training in school psychology is designated by master's (MA, MS) degrees and educational specialist degrees (EdS); this variation occurs by state and can be confusing. Noteworthy is that some master's degrees in school psychology contain approximately 60 credits, similar to the EdS degree. Some states make an additional designation available for those whose master's degree is granted at the 60-credit level to distinguish these from the 30-credit master's degree. Fortunately, only a few states credential school psychology practice with a 30-credit master's degree; this is not the norm and we will not address this level of practice. To reduce

There are two levels of training in school psychology: specialist and doctoral. Specialists typically have an education specialist degree (EdS) or a 60-credit master's.

the complexity in this discussion, the two levels of training in school psychology will be referred to as specialist (EdS degree or 60-credit master's) and doctoral.

School Psychology Training Is Both Broad and Specific

The task of training school psychologists involves providing a theoretical and scientific knowledge base as well as an array of professional practice skills. The knowledge base includes child development, principles of learning and behavior, personality development, social development, biological foundations, statistics, psychometric theory, and research. Course work is designed so that the foundational information comprises roughly a third of the training program. The remaining two-thirds are devoted to professional practice skills such as psychoeducational assessment, interviewing and counseling, consultation, intervention development, and the field placements that comprise practicum and internship. Three full-time faculty members who are appropriately trained and credentialed in school psychology and are active in the field of school psychology are the norm for accredited training programs, as is a commitment by the program to diversity.

Because training at the specialist level provides students with the necessary and sufficient credential for school-based practice, there is considerable similarity across training programs. Another reason for the similarity is program accreditation. Accreditation is an important process that assures that a program has clearly defined objectives and maintains conditions under which these goals can be achieved; self-study and review are important elements of the accreditation process. The requirements are somewhat more prescribed at the specialist level than at the doctoral level, as reflected in the training standards issued by the National Association of School Psychologists, (NASP, 2000b). A third reason for similarity across programs is the ongoing growth of the knowledge and practice base, yet many specialist programs try to remain at 60 credits.

The NASP standards require training programs to demonstrate that students have had course work and practical hands-on experience in 11 domains: (1) data-based decision making and accountability, (2) consultation and collaboration, (3) effective instruction and development of cognitive/academic skills, (4) socialization and development of life skills, (5) student diversity in development and learning, (6) school and systems organization, policy development, and climate, (7) prevention, crisis intervention, and mental health, (8) home/school/community collaboration, (9) research and program evaluation, (10) school psychology practice and development, and

(11) information technology. NASP approves programs, and accreditation is given by its partner, the National Council for the Accreditation of Teacher Education Programs (NCATE). Program accreditation is at both the specialist and doctoral levels.

Other requirements for accreditation of specialist programs by NASP/NCATE are a planned sequence of course work of at least 60 credits taken over 3 years, and a 1,200-hour internship, 600 hours of which must be in a public school. Interns are to receive at least 2 hours of supervision per week. For doctoral programs, the course work requirements are for 90 credits of graduate study over a minimum of 4 years, greater depth in course work than is typical for a specialist program, a 1,500-hour internship, and a doctoral dissertation. In the accreditation process, program resources, materials, procedures, and policies are reviewed. The report of evaluation of the program by the faculty must be performance-based in that the knowledge and skills of students must be systematically assessed as well as the impact of interns and graduates on the field. Quantifiable data are needed to meet this requirement, which in effect requires programs and internship sites to adopt the response-to-intervention (RTI) paradigm, irrespective of local practice, as is permitted by federal regulations. Student scores on the PRAXIS National School Psychology Exam developed by the Educational Testing Service must be provided. Not all states require this exam for practice as a school psychologist.

The additional course work in doctoral programs compared to specialist programs provides some latitude in training while permitting the program to meet accreditation standards. Doctoral programs are also accredited by the American Psychological Association (APA). Although there are course requirements that are generic for doctoral programs, the APA standards permit programs to define themselves and then demonstrate that the program has indeed met those standards. Should a doctoral program desire accreditation by both APA and NASP/NCATE, it must meet two sets of standards. In contrast to the APA requirements, the NASP standards (2000b) are more rigid in terms of content and the training sequence. For NASP/NCATE, the difference in training between the specialist level and the doctoral level is largely in the research training that occurs at the doctoral level. Doctoral programs may also contain courses in psychotherapy, school administration, neuropsychology, and so forth that are not typically available at the specialist level.

Accreditation of programs in professional psychology by the American Psychological Association (APA) is at the doctoral level only. In this process, the program seeking accreditation must submit a self-study that includes training goals, objectives, and practices. Information on students, faculty, and financial resources as well as program policies and procedures is included. The competencies students are expected to obtain and the outcome data that demonstrates the achievement of these competencies are provided. Other requirements include course work in generic requirements for professional psychology, such as developmental psychology and history and systems of psychology, and a 1-year internship. The supervising psychologist at the internship site must be licensed as a psychologist.

Impact of Accreditation Requirements

School psychology programs, similar to other programs in professional psychology, are expected to provide the education to qualify students for the necessary practice credentials and to meet the standards for education and training set forth by accrediting bodies. Institutions that train school psychologists at both levels typically have the specialist program embedded within the doctoral program. Thus, the task of the program director can be daunting in that the program should meet multiple sets of standards (that do not fully overlap) and must be sufficiently flexible to change as appropriate when new legislation and the accompanying regulations can result in changes in practice that are incorporated in training. Last, programs are often crafted to be unique in some way.

The impact of accreditation requirements therefore results in a curriculum at least partially prescribed, making it increasingly difficult to include all of the necessary training and experience within 60-credit specialist programs. Moreover, the data collection required for accreditation and its analysis require considerable faculty time. Accordingly, it is not uncommon for contemporary specialist programs to exceed 60 credits (the current average is about 72 credits). Not only does this make training more costly and lengthier but it can also limit what is taught. Additionally, it raises the question of whether training should be only at the doctoral level. Programs are often forced to balance providing students with a contemporary education, meeting accreditation standards, and offering the education and training in the skills most commonly used in the field. Practice in the field understandably lags behind what researchers are advocating, and a major way for potential practitioners to learn about promising new research is through their training programs. Program faculty need to teach what is contemporary; if contemporary and newer research-based information and practices are not taught in the training program, the prospective school psychologist may not learn this information. How can practitioners decide whether a specific technique or theory would be helpful in their practice if they have not been thoroughly introduced to it? Remember that being a reflective practitioner includes ultimately deciding how one will practice!

Another challenge to program faculty is deciding the extent to which they will incorporate their own specialty areas of knowledge and practice into the program. Faculty may also have strong beliefs as to which basic skills should be taught. With so much information to cover, teaching should be efficient to avoid duplication (as opposed to reteaching to reinforce skills) and the curriculum should be frequently reviewed and updated as appropriate. This task is more challenging for specialist programs than for doctoral programs for two reasons: the limited number of credits and the greater number of students in the specialist programs. The additional course work in doctoral programs may allow the inclusion of more specialized training or, at the least, introduction to such areas of practice (e.g., neuropsychology).

Challenges for Teaching

The knowledge base and practice of school psychology continue to grow, making it increasingly difficult to be a general practitioner who is fully competent in *all* skills. The growth of psychological testing is a case in point. The kinds and numbers of tests in common use have increased markedly over the last 30 years. It is no longer the norm for most school psychologists to use a similar battery of tests for the majority of referrals. Consequently, the growing repertoire of available tests means that programs are either going to be selective as to which tests they teach or allocate more instructional time to teaching testing. Moreover, test interpretation and diagnostics have become more sophisticated and complex, paralleling the advances in test construction and the emphasis on theoretical underpinnings in contemporary measures (see chapter 3 for a discussion).

Although the focal points of psychological assessment in school psychology are cognitive and achievement tests, school psychologists also assess the skills and processes of learning and social-emotional or personality assessment, as evaluation by these domains is required by law when a youngster is evaluated for the possibility of special education services. Because the assessment role of a school psychologist is more than simply being an "IQ tester," he or she needs adequate instructional time in the evaluation of other domains of functioning, particularly the social-emotional and personality domains. Indeed, the explanation for a child's poor academic functioning can be related to social-emotional and personality factors, even if the concerns in this area are at subclinical levels. Because it is not uncommon for school psychological referrals to be based on attentional or motivational factors, it would be remiss not to instruct future school psychologists in assessment practices that appropriately rule in or rule out these possibilities.

A domain that receives less attention (possibly because of an already full curriculum) is social-emotional and personality assessment. There could be several reasons for this lack of attention; many psychologists believe that (1) the multiple-rater questionnaires that are in extensive use today will always constitute a complete assessment; (2) the social-emotional aspects of functioning can be assessed by interview, observation, and historical review; and (3) the controversy surrounding the psychometric properties and empirical support of instruments considered projective tests renders these measures less worthy of the limited instructional time. This is unfortunate because school psychologists may be seen by other professional psychologists as professionals who are trained to conduct a thorough assessment when faced with more complex and challenging cases, yet fail to do so, despite having training in developmental disorders and psychopathology that makes them the ideal individuals to identify such problems in the nascent stages. Recent literature (Dana, 2007; Esquivel & Flanagan, 2007; Flanagan, 2007; Flanagan & Esquivel, 2006; Flanagan & Motta, 2007; Hughes, T. L., et al., 2007; Teglasi, 2007; Teglasi, Simcox, & Kim, 2007) provides direction for incorporating social-emotional and personality assessment into school psychology practice in ways that are consistent with theory and empirical data.

Counseling (and psychotherapy) is an area of school psychology practice that may not receive the amount of attention needed within the constraints of the curriculum. School psychologists clearly build skills in these practice areas through years of experience—for which there is *no* substitute—but the training program is responsible for the daunting tasks of familiarizing students with a number of types of counseling, teaching them how to interview, teaching them about theoretical principles that are operative in a therapeutic relationship (for a discussion, see chapter 5), and providing some hands-on experience using specific counseling techniques/modalities.

Another challenge for training programs is the development of cultural competence. School psychologists are more likely than other types of psychologists to have contact with individuals from a wide array of cultures because the primary employment setting is a public school. One precursor to cultural competence is realizing that there are numerous differences among cultures, many of which may not be apparent to those who are not members of the culture. The numbers of different cultures that may be common in particular locales add to the complexity of this task. In attempting to provide culturally competent services, the school psychologist must be aware that language, customs, etiquette, values, socioeconomic circumstances, and the structure of the family and family members' roles within the unit are just some of the variables determining whether the services will be acceptable to the client. An important job of the training program is to help students realize that the development and maintenance of cultural competence in practice is a never ending learning task.

An ongoing challenge for program faculty is to monitor the field for changing trends so as to anticipate when curriculum adjustments and changes might be needed. A recent example is the trend in the field toward the response-to-intervention (RTI) paradigm. Although RTI has not achieved universal acceptance, its use is sufficiently widespread that programs have needed to make changes, teaching more information on academic interventions along with the skills needed to track progress in systematic ways. Many programs are teaching traditional psychoeducational assessment as well as the theory and skills needed to work in an RTI environment.

Clearly, the training challenges are greater in specialist programs because of less training time and fewer credits in the curriculum. Although a substantial portion of the additional credits in doctoral programs is allocated to research/dissertation, there is also more room to teach a broader number of skills and theories than is possible in a 60-credit program.

Training for Varied Career Paths

Similar to other areas of professional psychology, school psychology can have varied career paths. At the specialist level, most individuals are practicing in public school settings; these are generally jobs that pay well and follow the school calendar. Conditions of employment are similar to those of teachers, including the benefits of belonging to a collective bargaining unit. Positions are also available at private schools and preschools; most of these positions serve special education populations. Some school psychologists find that they are interested in school administration; with the appropriate credentialing, school psychologists can become administrators of pupil services, school principals, and so forth. A career option for school psychologists that provides some flexibility is to work as an employee of an agency contracted by the respective state to provide special education-related school psychological services; the children receiving the services attend schools that often do not have a psychologist as a regular employee. Other possible employment settings are typically governmental entities, such as state hospital systems that serve children with psychiatric diagnoses.

Those trained at the doctoral level have more career options. Although career ladders are not available for school psychologists in school-based positions because these do not differentiate responsibilities between those who are at the specialist level versus those who are at the doctoral level, the doctorate may facilitate movement to administrative ranks, or make it possible for one to have employment as a psychologist secondary to the school-based position. Should a doctoral-level school psychologist pursue licensure as a psychologist, career options such as independent practice are possible. Hospital and clinic settings that rely on insurance reimbursement for some of the cash flow are also possible work settings for those who are licensed. Those at the doctoral level may also find secondary employment as adjunct faculty in university training programs; individuals with considerable experience as practitioners have something to contribute to school psychology training. The expertise of such individuals for practicum courses is a valuable asset to a training program.

Careers in academia and research settings are also options for those with a doctoral degree. If the academic position is within a school psychology training program, the individual should be certified as a school psychologist and licensed as a psychologist. This is important on two counts: it is desirable for training program faculty to have had some experience as practitioners and program faculty should be appropriately credentialed to supervise the services that are provided by students in the training program. Such positions are often housed within schools of education, although some are housed within arts and sciences-based psychology departments. The requirements for promotion and tenure are similar to those of all the faculty and include teaching, scholarship, and service. Environmentally, the day-to-day work experience is likely to be different if most colleagues are education professionals rather than psychologists. There is an ongoing shortage of school psychology faculty.

This array of career options means that training should include instruction and practice with a broad spectrum of practice skills. Training should also include an understanding of how psychologists function in other settings so as to facilitate referrals. This is important because school psychologists are often the first mental health professionals to come in contact with problems, yet the constraints of the setting in which they typically work does not permit them to be equipped to treat all problems of youth. Research training is important for all school psychologists as it prepares them to read the empirical literature with understanding, to apply research skills to evaluate interventions systematically, and to contribute to the empirical knowledge base of the field by conducting research.

Training to Develop Complex Integrated Skills

School psychologists are at least in theory full-service providers. Referring back to the archival description of school psychology (American Psychological Association, retrieved March 20, 2009, from www.indiana.edu/~div16/goals.html#archival), it is evident that a great number of professional functions and competencies fall within the purview of professional school psychology. Because school psychologists are full-service providers, they need to be skilled in multiple practice domains. Moreover, school psychologists often provide multiple services to the same clients, most commonly in succession. Thus, the notion of developing a niche practice is not necessarily a practical option for a school psychologist opting to be employed in the public schools.

Among the routine services that may be provided by school psychologists are psychoeducational assessment, consultation, counseling, and intervention development; most service activities would fall under one of those categories. Each of these activities has multiple components that vary across referral situations. Moreover, it is not uncommon for a school psychologist to have consulted with teachers to help a particular child, and then to develop an academic or behavioral intervention. Even more common is a sequence of consultation, intervention development, psychoeducational assessment, and additional intervention development or special education placement. Teaching future school psychologists to deliver such an array of services and to do so in a manner that encourages the use of data from one service to conduct the subsequent service is a challenging task, as students tend to view practice activities as discrete. This task is more challenging at the specialist level because there is less time in the training program to accomplish this goal, and training at the specialist level does not necessarily result in the same depth of conceptualization or broad use of resources in creative ways that occurs at the doctoral level. This is one distinction between the specialist level and the doctoral level.

Teaching students to think critically about what they are doing and to demonstrate appreciation for the rationales of what they are doing is challenging because students approach their assignments as course work, when the mindset that is needed is that the task is a professional service (that has a basis in established theory and empirical data) as opposed to a school assignment. Unfortunately, this way of thinking can be reinforced because the schools where most school psychologists will ultimately work tend to have forms that are completed for tasks such as updated psychoeducational assessments and functional behavioral assessments as well as behavior intervention programs.

Students learn of this and generally prefer that their course work requirements mirror the requirements of school buildings. From an instructional point of view, this is not necessarily the wisest course; teaching in this way makes it considerably more difficult to teach students to reason about professional tasks and the data. While it is important for students to learn facts, one important ingredient of professional functioning is the ability to apply the knowledge to client problems.

Students can be prompted to think by emphasizing procedures and application rather than following a template. For written products, a model that illustrates what a final product might look like is good, but far better instruction is providing a list of steps to follow. Sometimes the number of steps is large, but requiring students to follow steps as these apply to the circumstances for their client requires thinking and application. The expectation for this skill set is basic at the specialist level and grows in depth and complexity at the doctoral level.

Students can be given assignments that require them to answer thought-provoking questions. The questions can emphasize the strengths and weaknesses of particular techniques or strategies or can require responses that compare methods. Also important are assignments that require students to provide the rationale for their decision making. All of these activities are ways to promote being a reflective practitioner. Alternatively, students can be required to critique their own work. A specific example will help illustrate this idea.

Because school psychology has been so closely associated with psychoeducational assessment, many stakeholders (consumers of school psychological services) often almost automatically request an evaluation when a youngster encounters difficulty of just about any variety. The evaluation provides test scores that indicate the child's level of functioning. If an intervention is needed, it still has to be developed. Assessment skills include test selection, the testing process, data interpretation, data integration, reporting, conferencing, and intervention planning and development, all of which are conducted within the guidelines set forth by the ethics codes. However, in the case of academic difficulty, perhaps the student's difficulty with math computation, a more informative path might be a consultation with the teacher to discuss the specific nature of the student's difficulty and the manner of instruction, all of which could lead to suggestions for a different approach to instruction. The skills needed include conferencing, task analysis, review of data, additional conferencing, intervention planning and development, and the evaluation of the intervention efforts, all conducted within the guidelines set forth by the ethics codes. The point is that the same problem could be addressed with psychoeducational assessment or with consultation. Students could be required to discuss the strengths and weaknesses of each approach for the referral question, the rationale for clinical decision making, and the ethical principles that come into play. The overall process simulates reflective practice.

Postdoctoral Training

The School Psychology Synarchy (now known as the School Psychology Specialty Council) was launched in part to draft guidelines for postdoctoral residencies in school psychology. This optional training to deepen and strengthen the practice competencies of doctoral-level school psychologists has several purposes: (1) to extend previously acquired expertise so this can become part of cohesive sets of interrelated areas of advanced competencies for service delivery in a specified context, or with a particular population or problem area; (2) to emphasize competencies that are given less emphasis at the doctoral level but are included within the domain of school psychology; and (3) to introduce emerging trends in the scientific knowledge base, theoretical frameworks, or professional practice.

The guidelines for postdoctoral residencies in professional psychology are available at www.apa.org/ed/accreditation/qrg_postdoc.html. It is considered desirable for those individuals who complete postdoctoral residencies that meet the Education and Training guidelines so developed to become board certified by the American Board of Professional Psychology (ABPP).

PART V

Foundational
Competencies

TEN

Common Ethical and Legal Challenges in School Psychology

The purpose of this chapter is to discuss the ethics codes that school psychologists are expected to follow irrespective of their level of educational attainment. Also explored are practice competencies and reflective practice while following ethical principles as well as the requirements of law and regulation.

Ethics generally refers to a system of principles of conduct that guides the behavior of an individual (Jacob & Hartshorne, 2007). Ethics develops out of concern for individuals and within the context of particular cultures and societies. Acceptable and unacceptable behaviors are defined by ethics. The behaviors addressed by ethics are varied and range from etiquette and social customs to professional behavior. The National Association of School Psychologists (NASP) defines ethics as the formal principles that elucidate the proper conduct of a professional school psychologist (NASP, 2000a). The American Psychological Association (APA, 2002) does not define ethics per se but rather provides direction to its members through a set of ethical principles and a code of conduct. Moreover, the APA makes a distinction between professional behavior and personal behavior, indicating that the ethics code applies to professional activities only.

Important to note is that standards of ethics and professionalism are not necessarily equivalent in *all* situations, although there is considerable overlap. For example, there is latitude in the choice of theoretical orientation that a psychologist chooses to follow; that is a professional decision. Yet there are standards for treatment of individuals that are defined by ethics; these apply regardless of theoretical orientation. Competence is one such standard that forms the foundation of professional activities (Barnett et al., 2007).

For a number of reasons, ethical conduct is more complex than following a set of codified rules. Ethics codes are imperfect, as they are composed of sets of principles and specific standards. Because ethics codes are developed for use across a range of situations, they are not always as clear as desired (e.g., Bersoff, 1994; Hughes, J. N., 1986). Often multiple ethical principles will apply in any given situation; the demand characteristics of the situation, and often the law, will determine which principle is the primary one to be considered as one develops a course of action (Jacob & Hartshorne, 2007). Ethics codes are periodically updated and revised; this process is often in response to situations that occur in practice for which more explicit direction is desirable. Sections of the most recent revision of *Ethical Principles of Psychologists and Code of Conduct* (APA, 2002), as these apply to school psychology, are a case in point (Flanagan, Miller, & Jacob, 2005). Ethical codes provide guidance for professional decision making whereas ethical conduct involves making choices based on knowledge, reasoning, and personal values (Jacob & Hartshorne, 2007).

School Psychologists Follow Two Ethics Codes

School psychologists should be familiar with the ethics codes of both the American Psychological Association (APA) and the National Association of School Psychologists (NASP).

The two major organizations that represent the professional interests of school psychologists each have their own set of professional ethics that set standards for professional behavior and decision making. Regardless of membership in APA or the National Association of School Psychologists (NASP), school psychologists should be thoroughly familiar with the ethics codes of both organizations. Moreover, knowledge of both codes may be expected in the work setting. A broad knowledge base of ethical principles and standards is likely to help psychologists anticipate and prevent ethical problems from arising and make sound choices when faced with ethically challenging situations (Jacob & Hartshorne, 2007). The National Association of School Psychologists' *Principles for Professional Ethics* (NASP, 2000a) and the American Psychological Association's *Ethical Principles of Psychologists and Code of Conduct* (APA, 2002) have points in common, but there are differences because the NASP code was developed for school psychologists only. The APA code was developed to guide the practice and behavior of a variety of professional psychologists, such as clinical, school, and counseling psychologists; consequently, it is broader. Moreover, psychology licensing boards use the APA code to guide their work.

The APA code also applies to psychologists whose work activity is other than professional service delivery, such as those who conduct research with animals. Important to note is that in regard to the practice of school psychology, both the APA and the NASP address a similar array of common practice situations (see Table 10.1). Both codes effectively codify standards for practice and professional behavior.

Competent Ethical Practice

The ethics codes apply to school psychologists working in various settings, such as schools, independent practice, clinics, hospitals, and universities. In addition, there are state and federal regulations that impact psychological practice, such as No Child Left Behind (NCLB, 2001), the Family Educational Rights and Privacy Act (FERPA, 1974) and the Health Insurance Portability and Accountability Act (HIPAA, 1996), in addition to laws that

TABLE 10.1 **Comparison of Ethics Codes Applicable to School Psychology Practice**

PRINCIPLES FOR PROFESSIONAL ETHICS (NASP, 2000A)	ETHICAL PRINCIPLES OF PSYCHOLOGISTS AND CODE OF CONDUCT (APA, 2002)
Introduction	Introduction
	Preamble
Professional Competency	General Principles; Beneficence and Non-Malfeasance; Fidelity and Responsibility; Integrity; Justice Respect for People's Rights and Dignity Standard 2. Competence Standard 7. Education and Training,
Professional Relationships: Students; Parents; Legal Guardians; Surrogates; Community; Other Professionals; School Psychologist Trainees and Interns	Standard 1. Resolving Ethical Issues Standard 3. Human Relations Standard 4. Privacy and Confidentiality
Professional Practices Advocacy; Service Delivery; Assessment and Intervention; Reporting Data and Conference Results; Use of Materials and Technology; Research, Publication and Presentation	Standard 8. Research and Publication Standard 9. Assessment Standard 10. Therapy
Professional Practice Settings— Independent Practice Relationships with Employers; Service Delivery; Announcements /Advertising	Standard 5. Advertising and Other Public Statements Standard 6. Record Keeping and Fees

are to be followed. An important component of competent practice is the school psychologist's ability to negotiate the complex array of demands from various stakeholders while following regulatory and legal expectations. The complexity of a practice situation and its management often vary by setting.

The APA Ethics Code and School Psychology

The APA's Ethics Code, as it applies to school psychology, is deconstructed and examined here to illuminate the issues important to ethical decision making and practice behaviors of competent school psychologists. Those who desire more detail are urged to review the entire code.

INTRODUCTION AND APPLICABILITY

School psychologists are specifically mentioned as being expected to adhere to the code; this is new to the current code (Flanagan et al., 2005). The code is applicable in many situations and contexts. Possible activities relevant to school psychology are research, teaching, supervision, public service, policy development, social intervention, development of assessment instruments, conducting assessments, educational counseling, program design, and evaluation and administration. These activities can occur in person, or via mail, telephone, Internet, and other electronic contexts. This is a wide range of potential activities; most school psychologists can be competent in some. It is a most challenging and possibly unrealistic task to maintain up-to-date knowledge and skills in all the domains simultaneously. Thus, some practitioners may be capable in many of these areas over the course of their careers; a school psychologist who functions in this broad manner would be a lifelong learner, an attribute associated with competency.

PREAMBLE

School psychologists work to increase the science and professional practice bases of the specialty. This permits school psychologists to improve the condition of children, adolescents, families, and other school psychologists. The principles and standards provide direction for many situations concerned with the welfare and protection of individuals. This set of evolving ethical standards requires a lifelong effort by the practitioner to act ethically and encourage similar behavior in colleagues, including trainees. When new knowledge becomes available, school psychologists have a personal commitment to bring this to their clients with the overarching aim of improving their clients' condition. Using new knowledge in this manner is one way to be an advocate for clients. This variety of advocacy is leadership within the specialty, and another indicant of competence. Noteworthy is that the NASP (2000a) code specifically addresses the issue of advocacy.

GENERAL PRINCIPLES

The five General Principles (see sidebar) are not enforceable ethical standards but important values. These principles have a clear connection to school psychology practice and research.

Beneficence and non-malfeasance are shown by having consideration for and safeguarding the welfare of those with whom psychologists work professionally. This pertains to work in a number of domains that include professional practice and scholarship activities. School psychologists routinely work with vulnerable populations as practitioners and researchers. School psychologists work to avoid misuse use of their influence.

> **Five General Principles**
> 1. Beneficence and non-malfeasance
> 2. Fidelity and responsibility
> 3. Integrity
> 4. Justice
> 5. Respect for people's rights and dignity

In their professional relationships, school psychologists show fidelity and responsibility. Relationships are based on trust and acting in the best interests of stakeholders. In following standards of conduct, school psychologists are aware of their professional and scientific responsibilities and work to serve the best interests of those they work with. This can be particularly complex for school psychologists because there are numerous stakeholders: the child, the child's parents, the child's peers, the child's teachers, other school personnel, and the broader school community. School psychologists show integrity by promoting honesty, accuracy, and truthfulness in professional practices and science.

Integrity in school psychology practice means that school psychologists will be truthful, and if deception is part of approved research, there is adequate debriefing of research participants to correct misconceptions. Justice and fairness in school psychology practice means that all have access to and can benefit from school psychological services, with equal quality available for all. Respect for people's rights and dignity means that school psychologists provide safeguards for the rights and welfare of vulnerable populations and respect rights to privacy, confidentiality, and individual choice. This principle applies in most professional practice activities of school psychologists, as considerable work is with vulnerable, and possibly marginalized, populations. Vulnerable populations include youth in general, and more specifically, those who are being evaluated for, or are already placed within, the special education system, and those whose first language is not English, among others.

ETHICAL STANDARDS

The APA ethics code is composed of 10 standards, which contain subsections. For the exact details of the code, the reader is referred to the source document (APA, 2002). Important to remember is that school psychology is unique among the professional practice areas because *most* practice situations involve multiple stakeholders, whether it is parent and child, child and teacher, or others. The standards embodied in the code apply equally to all professional interactions in which the school psychologist engages. Thus, practice is more complex as compared to other practice areas, such as clinical psychology. The areas covered by the 10 Ethical Standards are (1) resolving ethical issues, (2) competence, (3) human relations, (4) privacy and confidentiality, (5) advertising and public statements, (6) record keeping and fees, (7) education and training, (8) research and publication, (9) assessment, (10) therapy.

Resolving Ethical Issues   In keeping with the first standard, school psychologists work to resolve conflicts between ethical standards and the expectations and practices of other settings, most commonly, the school setting. For school psychologists, who are employees of school systems, as well as those who consult as independent practitioners, situations may arise in which school employees, such as teachers, may not be bound to quite the same standards. At times, this can be misinterpreted by school personnel, who generally view school psychologists who are employees as teachers (see chapter 1 for a discussion) and professional equals. School psychologists explain that the standards are different (rather than "higher") and work within those standards to produce a result that is acceptable for all involved. This may similarly occur when legal requirements conflict with the ethics code. While school psychologists work to resolve such differences, if the dilemmas cannot be resolved, it is permissible to follow the law. This last point is new to the current version of the code (Flanagan et al., 2005; Knapp & VandeCreek, 2003).

Competence   Competence in practice is the second standard. Competence is a complex concept because it often comes into play in conjunction with other ethical principles. For example, competence is an aspect of assessment skills, therapy skills, working with diverse populations, teaching, and in the decision making that occurs when delegating work to others and supervising them. School psychologists have training and experience appropriate to the work they are conducting, and they are aware of the boundaries, or limits, of their training. When determining and expanding the boundaries of professional practice, the education and training to date are considered and additional education and training is sought as appropriate. Education and training vary from an organized course of study to supervision and consultation with other professionals. Because the expansion in professional knowledge is increasing at an exponential rate, the task is daunting. Moreover, it is not realistic to expect a professional psychologist to be competent in all practice techniques/situations/problems/populations in his or her specialty area. Nevertheless, maintaining competency is an ongoing effort. This is a particular problem for school psychology because the school psychologist who is an employee of a school district is theoretically expected to be able to provide some level of service to all the children in the building. The potential array of referral concerns is large. For this reason in particular, training in crisis intervention is an important component of graduate training in school psychology.

Particular concerns for school psychologists are working with diverse populations, receiving training on the newest versions of psychological tests, and so forth. The range of diverse populations is broad (see chapter 11 for a discussion). For school psychologists, it is possible that their graduate training program did not provide training in psychotherapy. Thus, to provide that service, the practitioner should undertake the appropriate training. Another appropriate option is to refer the individual to another professional psychologist, and for school psychologists who are school-based employees, to maintain a supporting role, so as to facilitate the needed communication and provide concrete support for the intervention, with the school setting. School psychologists also adopt this course of action if there is a personal problem or conflict that limits their ability to provide competent service.

An area of particular concern for school psychologists is working with linguistic minorities. This domain is highlighted because increasing numbers of linguistically diverse youth are in the nation's schools. School psychologists are often called upon to determine the nature of learning issues, which can range from the language barrier as the primary concern to learning and familial issues that are further complicated by a language barrier. Happily, the current edition of the APA code includes direction to school psychologists that provide greater clarity in these situations (Flanagan et al., 2005).

Several issues come into play when a child whose first language is not English is presented to the school psychologist; the issues relate to communication in the first place, and psychological testing. Regarding communication, if the child is unable to communicate in English, the most desirable option is to seek the help of a bilingual school psychologist. An alternative is to utilize an interpreter (e.g., Lopez, 2002); however, the interpreter must be trained and must be trustworthy and observe confidentiality. If the referral proceeds to the point that psychological testing is considered, there is increased complexity; this is addressed in greater detail in the discussion of the ethical standard on assessment.

Human Relations   An important part of human relations is to avoid doing harm and to minimize it when it cannot be avoided. School psychologists do not knowingly engage in harassment or discrimination. As school psychologists can have considerable power in their relationships with various stakeholders, they guard against potential exploitation of individuals who are clients and supervisees. Obtaining informed consent for psychological services or research is an important related concept. School psychologists guard against entering into relationships that limit their ability to act objectively. Potentially problematic are multiple relationships between a school psychologist and another individual that involve professional and personal components. Such relationships are to be avoided if they impair the school psychologist's objectivity, competence, or effectiveness in functioning as a psychologist. Moreover, relationships that potentially exploit or harm the other individual are to be avoided. Multiple relationships that fall outside of these criteria are acceptable.

Should a school psychologist be in a situation in which a potentially harmful multiple relationship arises, he or she should take steps to resolve the situation in a manner consistent with the code. Should a multiple relationship be the result of a legal proceeding, the psychologist should clarify the relationship to all parties from the beginning. In a related vein, relationships that involve potential conflicts of interest are to be avoided, particularly when these may cause harm or exploit individuals. Relationships with other professionals are important; school psychologists cooperate with other professionals as appropriate.

Because school psychologists are often functioning as employees rather than independent practitioners, they are providing services through an organization. For example, a psychological evaluation that is provided under the auspices of a school is conducted on different terms from one that is provided in an independent practice situation. The use of the data, which individuals have access to the data, and the limits of confidentially need to be clarified to avoid misunderstandings. If a school psychologist is employed by a legal entity such as the prison system, special explanations are needed to ensure the incarcerated individual understands that the school psychologist's client is the prison system.

The NASP Code (2000a) addresses specific concerns that apply to school psychologists who work in multiple settings. Should a school psychologist be a school employee and an independent practitioner, referrals of children who reside within the school district of employment, including the non-public schools, is prohibited. Such a standard makes sense for the school psychologist as well as the stakeholders. The children continue to obtain services through the school district (which is also required to provide the services that fall under special education to those in nonpublic schools), and the school psychologist avoids situations that are awkward at the least. If the child who is in need of services is not eligible for services from the school district because he or she did not meet special education criteria, the school psychologist assists the family by advising them of other sources where they can obtain the needed services.

Privacy and Confidentiality   School psychologists respect the rights of stakeholders to privacy and maintain confidentiality. School psychologists practicing independently do not communicate with third parties without permission from the child's parents. For school psychologists who are employees of school systems, the standard is more complex. Clearly, there is no communication with third parties external to the school system without parental permission. Within the school system, the limits of confidentially generally rely upon the principle of legitimate educational interest, which often means that the child's teacher or the school principal routinely has access to the information. It is important that this point is made clear to the child's parents before services are provided. In the interest of privacy, the information contained in written and electronic records should be limited to that which is essential to understand the case. This point is even more important in school settings because access to written reports is granted to those with legitimate educational interests.

Because it is common to consult with other professional psychologists about cases, information that could identify a client is shared only if prior permission from the client was granted. Similar care is taken when material is used for teaching purposes.

Advertising and Other Public Statements   School psychologists who provide services independently, those who are university faculty, and those who offer continuing education workshops are more typically concerned with this standard than those school psychologists who are employed within school systems. The key point is accuracy and the presentation of truthful information that is not deceptive; claims made about procedures or services must be realistic.

The truthfulness in information applies to statements about services provided by professional psychologists as well as the representation of their credentials and professional affiliations. Fees for services are represented accurately. Degrees that are claimed as a basis for providing services are noted only if obtained from a regionally accredited institution and are included in the basis for licensure. Claims about the effectiveness of a particular service or research findings are accurate and realistic. Statements made in legal proceedings are accurate. Brochures that describe training programs and workshops are accurate as they relate to presenters, learning objectives, and fees.

Psychologists who engage others to prepare advertisements retain responsibility for the accuracy and truthfulness of such statements. Statements made to the media are based on professional knowledge and represent current practice standards; there is no indication of a professional relationship with the media. Testimonials are not permitted from current or prior patients. Solicitation of clients for service is not permitted as the populations are vulnerable; contacts that provide additional appropriate services for those already in treatment or to provide for those in disaster situations are appropriate. School psychologists practicing in school settings commonly provide services on a crisis basis; the services are often to determine the extent to which the identified problem requires intervention. The psychologist then determines whether the problem can be addressed adequately within the school setting or whether there should be a referral for professional services outside the school building. One of the most common situations in which this might occur is when a youngster expresses suicidal ideation.

Record Keeping and Fees   Professional services and research data are properly documented; in addition to serving as an official record, this permits other professionals to continue work when the psychologist who documented the professional services or research data is no longer seeing the client or working on the project. For those providing services as employees of school systems or other agencies, institutional guidelines are followed. For those working independently, billing records are accurate. Treatment records are subject to confidentiality. In school settings, only those with a legitimate educational interest may have access to the records; in other settings, parallel procedures need to be in place. Independent practitioners and those working in a mental health setting other than schools follow HIPAA (1996) guidelines for the security of records. School-based records are subject to the FERPA (1974) requirements. Researchers who enter data into electronic systems code the data so it is not personally identifiable. Raw data that contain personally identifiable information are maintained securely. When psychologists leave practice, they develop plans for the security and transfer of their records.

For school psychologists providing services on a fee-for-service basis, fees are accurately represented and the billing procedures are consistent with law. Should it become apparent that a client will have difficulty paying for services, referral is made to an appropriate source that is financially affordable for the client. Adjustments to the fee can be made for exceptional circumstances should there be no appropriate source for referral, so as to maintain access to services. Collection agencies or legal means are not used unless the client is informed and there has been opportunity for him or her to make prompt payment. Records are not withheld for nonpayment of fees. Bartering arrangement with patients is acceptable in some limited circumstances; it is important to consider the multiple relationships involved, and the details of the bartering arrangement must be clear from the outset.

Education and Training   Similar to other domains of ethical practice, those who are faculty in school psychology training programs are expected to be accurate in teaching and the description of training programs. Moreover, training programs should meet current standards and provide the education and training that is needed for students to obtain certification as a school psychologist, to be eligible to enter doctoral programs, and to gain licensure as a psychologist. The training experience for school psychologists should be an organized set of didactic courses and field experience. Students are made aware of how they are evaluated at the beginning of academic courses or supervision; they receive feedback on their performance on a regular basis.

Students are not required to disclose personal information unless it is a written program requirement that was made known as part of the admissions requirements or if it is clearly necessary to determine whether personal issues are negatively impacting the student's ability to meet requirements and provide supervised services to others. If therapy is part of program requirements, students are provided with a list of providers who are not affiliated with the program.

Research and Publication   Although most school psychologists are practitioners, some practitioners conduct research. Research is conducted
under conditions of institutional approval and informed consent from
participants. Because school psychology research often involves children,
parental permission and assent from the child is required. Essential is the
protection of participants from harm. Participants who are graduate students, or other subordinates, also require extra care. Care must be taken to
prevent adverse consequences should prospective participants choose to
decline or withdraw from research participation. The psychologist should
make clear that the availability of school psychological services for youth
is not impacted by whether the child participates in the project or with-
draws from it. Data are reported accurately and publication credit is in
proportion to the individual's contribution to the effort. Data are shared
with other professionals for reanalysis. Journal reviewers respect intellectual property rights.

Assessment   A major portion of school psychology practice is assessment
and activities related to the assessment process: for this reason, this standard receives particular attention here. Consistent with contemporary
practice, school psychologists base conclusions on data of sufficient quantity that the results can be substantiated. Tests are used in the manner for
which they were developed. Tests are interpreted in light of their reliability
and validity *or* for performance-based measures of personality for which
traditional psychometric concepts are not applicable (Anastasi, 1988) in
light of research and theory-based recommendations. Tests are administered in the client's preferred language or a language that the client is
competent in.

The 2002 version of the code addresses psychological evaluations of linguistic minorities with greater specificity than prior editions of the code.
The school psychologist must make certain that the data and interpretations are representative of the child's functioning. Linguistic and cultural differences introduce additional variables that increase the complexity of this
task. Although modern norming procedures result in measures that do not
have *systematic* bias, there are concerns with the use of current measures
because the translations of test items do not necessarily exhibit exact correspondence. Moreover, there may not be sufficient representation of individuals with the same background as the child in the norm group. This latter
point can occur with nonverbal measures as well. Should it be determined
that using an interpreter is desirable, permission is needed from the child's

parents, and the school psychologist must make it clear that that the interpreter is expected to maintain confidentiality.

The greatest practice-related difficulties occur when the child speaks some English and may even be able to have a conversation but lacks sufficient understanding of the language to handle an assessment adequately. Researchers have established that there are phases of second language acquisition as it relates to schooling (Cummins , 1984); an individual may acquire adequate conversational language skills in approximately 2 years, but up to 7 years are needed for him or her to have language adequate to manage the academic demands of schooling. Because academically related linguistic difficulties persist, it is wise to use the services of a bilingual school psychologist for interviewing and most certainly for psychological testing. School personnel are often unfamiliar with this information or do not accept it, and they are often reluctant to contract for a bilingual school psychologist. This creates an important advocacy role for the school psychologist; the NASP (2000a) code specifically mentions advocacy as an obligation of the school psychologist.

Testing occurs under conditions of informed consent. Parents must provide written permission for a child to be tested, and assent from the child is desirable. When the child agrees to testing, the psychologist is much more likely to be able to establish adequate rapport with him or her, and this rapport should lead to more representative test results as the child will be much more at ease and trusting. School psychologists conduct tests and interpret the data only if they have training and experience with the particular instrument. They use and draw conclusions from only data that are current. Because the useful life of a test is briefer than in the past, tests are now revised more frequently; this provides an additional responsibility on the school psychologist to obtain the necessary training and experience to utilize these new versions competently.

Ideally, test data are released only to other qualified individuals with the written permission of the client or the client's parent/guardian, in the case of a child. Clients, or the parents/guardian, if appropriate, may request the raw test data as per provisions of HIPAA (1996) and FERPA (1974). This introduces two considerations: one is test security, the other is misinterpretation of the data by those who are not trained to interpret it. For these reasons, it is wise for school psychologists to consider several ways of proceeding. Most stakeholders will not realize that test security is an issue but may appreciate that point when it is explained. Some stakeholders will be agreeable to receiving a written report and an explanation of it. It is also possible to ask such individuals if there is another qualified professional to whom the data may be released, as an acceptable resolution. The qualified professional is to be a psychologist who has the appropriate training and knowledge to interpret and explain the data to the parents, while protecting the security of test materials and guarding against misuse of the data. If not, however, the laws are such that the data are to be released. Worth noting is that interpretations made of IDEA (1997) led school administrators to decide that reports must be given to the child's parents as a matter of course because parents are entitled to have access to the information that led to educational decision making by IEP teams. A concern is that this has become routine practice regardless of whether parents request the data. In some locales, it is not uncommon for parents to receive a report in the mail in advance of any meeting with school professionals; this, of course is one way misinterpretation of the information can occur. It is clearly better to arrange a parent meeting before the parents receive a report on their child as a proactive way to limit misunderstandings and difficulties.

Therapy   The standards that apply to this principle will more often apply to school psychologists in independent practice and clinic settings, although there is some applicability in school settings. Similar to assessment practice, informed consent is obtained for therapy. For group or family therapy, consent should be obtained from all participants; additional attention must be paid to confidentiality and its limits. Particularly applicable to school-based practitioners is the treatment of youth already served by others and interruption of treatment. School psychologists practicing in schools communicate with practitioners serving the child outside of the school setting and take a supporting role. The interruption in treatment that occurs as a function of the school year may necessitate referral to an independent practitioner to provide continuity for the summer months.

Requirements of Law/Regulation

The laws that provide for and regulate the education of special populations may impact school psychology practice. This impact to school psychology will likely (but not necessarily) be greater in the school setting than it might be in independent practice. What is important here is that these public sector regulations impact schooling, irrespective of what a school psychologist might think is appropriate. This situation increases the complexity of decision making for school psychologists because of the possibility that what a professional school psychologist considers in the child's best interest is something other than what the school is willing or obligated by law to provide. Thus, it may also impact the manner in which a school psychologist communicates information to stakeholders about educational options and educationally related services (such as in school counseling). Moreover, it may indirectly impact the way information about out-of-school services (such as psychotherapy) is discussed. Not surprisingly, the APA code is silent on these issues; the NASP code provides some clarity and direction.

INDIVIDUALS WITH DISABILITIES EDUCATION ACT (IDEA)

The initial version of this federal law was passed in 1975 and was called the Education for Handicapped Children Act. The law has been revised (1986, 1997, 2002, 2004) in response to societal changes, changes in the school-age population, and periodic need to update and improve practices. This law provides for the education of youth with special needs, from the point of referral for assessment to the point at which services are no longer needed, or age 21, whichever is later. The remarks made about the IDEA are not intended to be exhaustive but to be examples of portions of the regulations that are more likely to directly involve school psychologists. Interested readers should consult the source documents, which are part of the Code of Federal Regulations (available at http://ecfr.gpoaccess.gov). A considerable part of the regulations are procedural safeguards; these roles for monitoring compliance with regulations are often charged to special educators who are also certified school administrators.

The changes in law and subsequent changes in state-level regulations address an array of matters, such as the classification scheme that is used to determine eligibility. The changes have been an expansion, such as the addition of laws and regulations that provide for preschool and infant services, and the addition of eligibility categories, such as traumatic brain injury. Refinements have also been made in the definitions of disabilities and eligibility criteria. Changes have occurred in the acceptance of parental decisions (when the school disagrees) that give parents the final decision-making power (Jacob & Hartshorne, 2007). Periodic changes in the scope and requirements of evaluation, reevaluation, and Individual Education Plans (IEPs) or their equivalents for youngsters aged birth to 2, which are called Individual Family Service Plans (IFSPs) have also occurred. Other changes in the law and regulations have occurred in response to practices involving racial/ethnic and linguistic minorities (Lambert, 1981); these changes have limited misdiagnosis and overidentification of students as educationally disabled. An additional welcome change is the availability of funding for assistance to youngsters for *early intervention services*; these services are not intended for those who are suspected of requiring special education (IDEIA, 2004) and may include counseling or behavioral interventions. Moreover, the law is now requiring that schools use scientific or empirically supported practices.

SECTION 504 AND THE AMERICANS WITH DISABILITIES ACT

These laws have far reaching implications outside of the school setting, as these are antidiscrimination acts. The implications for the schools are actually secondary to the original purposes.

Section 504   Section 504 of the Rehabilitation Act of 1973 may impact the professional activities of school psychologists. This law was initially intended to address the rights of handicapped youth in schools, yet it was in a secondary role relative to the Education for All Handicapped Children, the forerunner of the IDEA. Subsequent reviews of the law revealed that there are situations that may not fall under broader regulations and could be addressed by invoking the provisions of Section 504 (Jacob & Hartshorne, 2007). Essentially, youngsters may qualify for school-based services under this law rather than the IDEA, because there may be a medical diagnosis (e.g., attention-deficit hyperactivity disorder), but the extent of the difficulty is not sufficient to trigger eligibility for services under the IDEA. The services are often uncomplicated accommodations, such as extended time for examinations that are needed to otherwise maintain the youngster in a regular education program. The roles for school psychologists are generally in the areas of assessment, advocacy, and intervention planning.

Americans with Disabilities Act (ADA)   This act addresses accessibility for those who are disabled in settings that serve the public. For schools, the impact has been to have wheelchair accessible entrances to buildings and elevators. Compliance with the law involved construction in existing buildings.

NO CHILD LEFT BEHIND (NCLB)

This act increases accountability for school districts in that statewide standardized test scores must document yearly progress. Among the positives are increased attention given to the quality of education and the progress of minority students. The negatives include emphases on teaching to the test and limitations placed on the curriculum because there is an overriding emphasis on raising test scores. Perhaps more important, the act represents a change in thinking in that children are now required to meet increased standards as opposed to minimum standards of competency. The increased standards are not necessarily appropriate for all youngsters, as modifications have been made to the standards that must be met for those who are educationally disabled.

ELEVEN

Individual and Cultural Diversity Considerations

Diversity, in all of its forms, influences school psychology in numerous ways. School psychologists need to keep abreast of research and current practice recommendations as a precondition to culturally competent practice. The influence of diversity is profound, impacting the manner in which concerns are conceptualized, whether an intervention is offered and accepted, and the type and extent of intervention made available. Moreover, current thinking and professional literature has adopted an increasingly broad conceptualization of diversity. Thinking and practice in regard to diversity issues has changed markedly since 1900 (Esquivel, Warren, & Olitzky, 2007); for example, thinking has progressed from the "melting pot" to a greater acceptance and promotion of diversity. The influence of diversity includes the identity of consumers of school psychological services, including children, teachers, parents, and school administrators; linguistic variety; and cultural variety. In this chapter, we address (1) educational influences and limitations, including linguistic diversity, bilingual education, special education, and gifted youth; (2) physical and other health limitations; (3) ethnic/cultural background; (4) sexual orientation; and (5) spirituality/religion. There is considerable variability and some overlap among and within these groupings.

School psychologists who are working in school settings may see more diversity in practice than any other type of psychologist. School psychologists do not choose their clients; they do not have the option of screening prior to an appointment, nor do they necessarily have the luxury of referring clients to other psychologists. School psychology is a service that is available in public schools, theoretically for all. Vane (1985) noted that school psychologists have more to do with the public than other types of psychologists and that one of the distinguishing features of school psychology is the variety it offers in practice. That variety we now call diversity. The information known about diverse groups of youth and their needs is applicable across many school psychological services, such as assessment, counseling, and consultation, and it is an important ingredient for culturally competent practice.

School psychologists working in school settings often are more exposed to diversity than other types of psychologists.

Educational Influences and Limitations

Culturally and linguistically diverse youth are often not achieving as well as their nonminority counterparts. Numerous influences can impact education both negatively as well as positively. Limitations come in a variety of forms that influence education and are found within youth belonging to minority and nonminority groups, including cognitive weaknesses, learning disorders, disorders such as autism, social-emotional concerns, linguistic barriers, limited opportunity, and socioeconomic variables. Some of these limitations may co-occur with considerations such as diversity in ethnic and cultural background. The explanation for why a particular child is encountering difficulty in school is often multiply-determined and complex. Many of the youth who are brought to the attention of school psychologists appear to have limitations in ability; often this is the reason for referral. Approximately 16% of all youth have a cognitive ability score on a standardized test that is at least one standard deviation below the mean (i.e., 85 and below). In contrast, approximately 16% of all youth earn scores on standardized measures of cognitive ability that is at least one standard deviation above the mean (i.e., 115 or higher); this, too, represents diversity.

Nevertheless, the explanation for limitations in measured ability can vary widely. It is also possible that what is measured as a limitation may not be a limitation so much as a manifestation of one of the variables that define diversity. One such variable is acculturation status. The process of acculturation or adapting to a new cultural environment may be contributing to a student's seeming limitations. Acculturation takes place in terms of environment, school, how things are done, and so forth. The process of acculturation is likely to be stressful; this is not necessarily unexpected (see Ryan-Arredondo & Sandoval, 2005), but ascertaining that acculturation stress definitely does or does not contribute to school-related problems may be difficult. Other sources of problems that appear to be limitations in ability are in fact linguistic differences, physical limitations, limited opportunities,

Acculturation can be a stressful process for children and can contribute to school-related problems.

and so forth; the point is that an ability measure may be assessing extraneous (but important) variables that negatively impact functioning, in addition to ability.

Linguistic Diversity

One of the most challenging issues for practicing school psychologists is addressing linguistic diversity appropriately. The implications for instruction are vast, although greater attention may be given to assessment issues, which will precede instructional issues. Nationally, the number of English Language Learners (ELLs) in public schools increased from over three million students in 1995–96 to over five million students in 2005–2006 (National Clearinghouse for English Language Acquisition, 2008). Estimates of the number of school psychologists capable of providing services in a language other than English show that the need far exceeds the supply. The directory of the National Association of School Psychologists (NASP) indicates that on October 14, 2008, 281 individuals identified themselves as bilingual school psychologists, less than 1% of the national membership. Miranda and Gutter (2002, p. 597) said of school psychology: "it appears unlikely that the field will attract a greater minority population in the next decade." Taking these facts together provides some indication of the magnitude of the concern.

Given the facts, it is evident that the task is potentially daunting for the few individuals who can provide services to linguistically diverse youth in the client's native language. Although some of these youth are immigrants, many were born in the United States; in such circumstances, the parents and/or a caregiver often have limited English proficiency and the youngster develops a primary linguistic proficiency in the native language of the caregiver. For some, the challenge does not end with the matter of learning English. Some youth have learning problems of varied origin reaching above and beyond English proficiency. It is also possible that they have a weak command of their native language. Only a bilingual evaluator could address that situation in an ethical and technically sound (to the point that evaluation tools permit) manner that separates and clarifies the issues. Moreover, for over 20 years we have known that it takes approximately 2 years to develop adequate conversational proficiency in a second language and 5 to 7 years to develop linguistic proficiency that is adequate for instructional purposes (Cummins, 1984).

There are very few bilingual school psychologists, making it difficult to provide services to linguistically diverse youth.

Thus, it is not uncommon to find a youngster who is conversational in English yet needs a bilingual evaluation to help determine whether his or her issues are command of a language or other learning issues. It is a situation that poses a challenge to school professionals, as it is sometimes necessary to expend effort convincing those who have administrative responsibility that a bilingual evaluator must be called upon. Not only do many school systems not have bilingual evaluators; they must deal with a wide range of languages. Major urban systems such as the New York City Department of Education have an in-house workforce to meet the needs of this population of youth.

Most locales (e.g., smaller suburban and rural districts) rely on obtaining the services contractually, through a cooperative. For example, according to the website, as of October 22, 2008, the Nassau County (New York) Board of Cooperative Educational Services provides bilingual psychological, educational, and speech/language evaluations in approximately 40 languages. The issues surrounding assessment of individuals whose first language is other than English are ethical (see Flanagan et al., 2005, for a discussion) and technical, representing a unique set of professional practice competencies. If ethical or technical issues are not fully considered in a particular situation, there is considerable risk of misdiagnosis, followed by inappropriate educational treatment recommendations and inappropriate instruction or instructional placement. A number of legal precedents have been set (see Jacob & Hartshorne, 2007, for a discussion) to provide procedural and practice safeguards for linguistic/racial/ethnic minority youth that have set standards and guide practice.

Racial/Ethnic Background and Learning

BILINGUAL EDUCATION

Cloud (2007) describes three types of programs for the education of bilingual youth: (1) English as a Second Language Programs (ESL) or a transitional bilingual education program, (2) maintenance bilingual education programs, and (3) two-way bilingual education programs. The manner in which instruction in the native language varies across the different types of programs is the defining issue. ESL programs focus upon learning English; content area instruction is secondary. For programs that aim to retain (and build) skills in the native language, instruction is geared to the participants' level of English proficiency (Baker, 2001). Despite the possibilities, ESL programs (or transitional programs) are the most common variety of bilingual program (Baker, 2001).

Bilingual education programs that foster bilingualism are typically time limited (Cloud, Genesee, & Hamayan, 2000), although students often remain in these programs longer than children remain in ESL programs. ESL programs, in contrast, typically aim to develop functional competencies in English that are defined by test-based exit criteria. A key issue is that the bilingual instruction be developmentally sensitive (Cummins, 1986) and permit continued learning in, and of, the native language. These programs focus on youngsters maintaining, strengthening, and learning two languages while progressing in the curriculum. Maintenance programs are for non-native speakers of English. Two-way bilingual education programs have a varied class composition in that there are youngsters whose native language is English and others whose native language is not English. The object is to train all youngsters in the class in the two languages (Cloud, 2007), as it has been identified that for these youngsters, in general, they fare better when the native language is maintained (Thomas, W. P., & Collier, 1998)

LANGUAGE AND ACADEMIC ACHIEVEMENT

Genesee, Lindholm-Leary, Saunders, and Christian (2005) reviewed the limited research available in refereed sources on the academic achievement of English language learners. The research they studied indicates that bilingual proficiencies and literacy are related to academic achievement in both languages. While this suggests that there may be developmental interdependencies across two languages, the data are largely correlational. This is congruent with prior research that consistently found educational performance to be better when youngsters were served in some form of a bilingual program, as opposed to ESL (e.g., Willig, 1985). Greene (1998) conducted a meta-analysis of 11 studies and reached similar conclusions; considerably more studies were excluded from the analysis due to methodological flaws. Despite empirical support, educational practice lags.

Diversity, Learning, and Academic Achievement   Kane and Boan (2005), in a review of multicultural learning styles, summarized key findings. The research on learning styles across African Americans, Asian Americans, Hispanic Americans, and Native Americans reveals an important finding. There is overlap across groups. No clear preferences were demonstrated among field-dependent, field-independent, kinesthetic, sensing, judging, auditory, peer-oriented/extroverted visual, sequential, and perceiving learning styles. Suggested instructional preferences include clear directions with concrete activities, use of manipulatives, step-by-step instructions, structured classrooms, interaction with teachers as reinforcement, small-group instruction, cooperative learning, independent/individual activities, visual stimuli, hand-on activities, flexible instruction, and visual stimuli emphasizing inter-relationships. It is fair to state that learning style and instructional prefer-ences will vary from child to child, independent of racial/ethnic background. Moreover, these preferred learning styles and instructional preferences are also commonly observed within the White majority population.

Keith and Fine (2005) proposed and tested a model to explain multicul-tural influences on school learning. Variables included in the model were ethnic and family backgrounds (White, Asian American, Hispanic, African American, Native American), previous achievement, quality of instruction, motivation, quantity of instruction, and grades. Each variable impacted learning across ethnic and family backgrounds, although the contribution of each variable to the end result varies. Continued achievement for Anglo Americans, African Americans, Hispanics, and those of Asian American descent was based on past achievement. Motivation and quality of instruc-tion are intermediary variables that exerted an impact on all groups except the Native Americans, for whom the model does not apply. Motivation has the greatest amount of impact upon grades for those of Anglo and Asian backgrounds; quality of instruction had the greater impact for African Americans and Hispanic students.

Although the literature discussed thus far does not support differences in learning that are explained by cultural influences and variables, there is appeal in the notion of providing learning opportunities in ways that may be culture specific. VanDerHeyden and Burns (2005) suggest that Cronbach's (1957) aptitude by treatment interactions provide a theoretical basis for this appeal. Yet, data indicate (Gresham, 2002; Gresham & Witt, 1997) that the aptitude by treatment interactions are not substantiated by the data in a num-ber of domains that include special education, neuropsychology, and cogni-tive processing. Given the facts, there is little reason to suspect that aptitude by treatment interactions would produce differentially superior results for those of culturally diverse backgrounds.

Effective instruction is critical to the school success of all youth, indepen-dent of race, ethnicity, and culture (VanDerHeyden & Burns, 2005). Effec-tive instructional practices are supported by empirical data. The ingredients of effective instruction are pacing, an adequately challenging curriculum, the effective use of instructional time, and teacher expectancies that chal-lenge rather than overwhelm the student. The data indicate that although individual differences explain many of the variations in individual achieve-ment, variables that impact education must be examined in combination, with each member of the school's team uniquely contributing to school effectiveness. Schools must be systematic in their practices by setting goals, collecting data, and truly evaluating the educational enterprise.

Special Education

The special education enterprise is populated with youngsters aged birth to 21 years whose measured cognitive ability is often below average. Important to note is that the limitations in cognitive ability contribute to the reasons a child might be referred for an evaluation to determine if he or she is eligible for special education, but those limitations are often not the sole reason. The student may have weaknesses in academic areas, difficulty learning, difficulties in the speech-language domains, difficulty paying attention, and social-emotional concerns, among other areas of difficulty. Youngsters aged birth to 2 (services offered in this period are sometimes referred to as early intervention), and ages 3 to 5 (preschool) are covered by state and federal regulations that are based on multiple classification systems that take development and schooling into account; these differ from those in the *Diagnostic and Statistical Manual of Mental Disorders, 4th Edition, Text Revision* (*DSM-IV-TR*, American Psychiatric Association, 2000), which describes and categorizes psychiatric disorders. The manner in which services are accessed and delivered varies by regulations that apply for the individual child's age (retrieved February 22, 2009, from http://idea.ed.gov/download/finalregulations.pdf).

A different set of federal regulations provides the classification system that applies to school-aged children (5–21) with disabilities (the implementation can vary across states) as those who evidence autism or have hearing impairments (including deafness), mental retardation, multiple disabilities, orthopedic impairments, other health impairments, serious emotional disturbance, specific learning disabilities, speech or language impairments, traumatic brain injury, and visual impairments including blindness (U.S. Department of Education, 2006). Also included are youngsters who have difficulty meeting the state standards for their current grade placement. In addition, some states follow supplementary guidelines for children aged 3 to 9 years that recognize developmental delays; these guidelines may help address the frequently unavoidable psychometric limitations (see Bracken, Keith, & Walker, 1998) in the tests that are often used to detect disabilities in young children, or may simply prevent smaller problems from becoming larger ones.

Thus, the range of youth who may be eligible for special education services is diverse; the characteristics of such youth span learning, social-emotional, and physical development, as well as health and wellness. The pedagogical techniques and both short-term and long-term expectations for these young-sters vary. The majority of youth placed in special education can function independently and be strong contributors to society. Other special education youth may have less optimistic prognoses for independence and the ability to contribute to society, and they more appropriately may be considered indi-viduals with special needs for the duration of their lives. Those youngsters' needs extend into adulthood and will impact their independent social func-tioning and employment. School psychologists provide direct services to this population, such as psychoeducational assessment and counseling. Indirect services, such as parent and teacher consultation, often focusing on instruc-tion and behavior (see chapter 7 for a discussion) are also among the services school psychologists provide. Ethical behavior on the part of school psychol-ogists includes advocacy, or assisting these individuals to obtain the services they need. There is a considerable literature available on special education beyond the scope of this book. Readers are directed to the *Encyclopedia of Special Education* (Reynolds & Fletcher-Janzen, 2007).

Gifted Youth

Although a very small segment of the population, gifted youth are a highly diverse group among themselves that may not receive needed attention. The theoretical base for giftedness has evolved, and definitions have been conse-quently modified. Reis and Renzulli (2004) indicate that recent work defines giftedness in terms of multiple aspects: high self-concept, motivation, and creativity (Siegler & Kotovsky, 1986), in addition to high cognitive ability, are included in the contemporary definitions. Nevertheless, Renzulli's (1978) definition that includes high levels of creativity and task commitment, in combination with high intellectual ability, remains pertinent. The federal definition of giftedness, based on the Jacob K. Javits Gifted and Talented Stu-dents Education Act of 1988 (retrieved October 18, 2008, from www.ed.gov/policy/elsec/leg/esea02/pg72.html) considers high performance and excep-tional potential in cognitive ability and academic aptitude as well as outstand-ing ability in visual and performing arts. Not all entities use this definition; some exclude the performing arts, and others include leadership and cre-ativity (e.g., Stephens & Karnes, 2000). There is recognition that educational programs or services beyond those normally provided by the regular school program are needed for such youth to realize their full potential. When using cognitive ability as the basis for giftedness, approximately 1% (cognitive abil-ity test score of 130 or more) of the population might be considered gifted, although high cognitive ability will not necessarily be a precondition to gift-edness in the arts (Oades-Sese, Esquivel, & Anon, 2007).

Gifted youth often have needs to be addressed apart from their unique abilities. Child development is not uniform across domains under typical (whatever that means) conditions; this is more pronounced for those who exhibit giftedness. The characteristics of the gifted are broad and vary across individuals. Learning can be deeper and more rapid, and in cognitive domains, gifted youth can be more similar to older youth. Memory and reasoning skills often outpace the skills of their age peers. In that regard, gifted youth may have better relationships with individuals older than themselves. Yet gifted youth often develop similarly to their age peers physically, socially, and emotionally. Moreover, they may have specific social-emotional concerns; thus the social-emotional and interpersonal needs of gifted youth can be complex. The social-emotional concerns of gifted youth are most often related to not fitting in with their peers, as their interests, personality, and vocabulary size often differ from those closest to them in age. Remember that children may be gifted in one domain but not in others, which may introduce additional complexity in their efforts to fit in comfortably with their peers. For example, a child may be gifted in regard to math concepts, yet have poor spelling skills, or weak social skills. Gifted youth tend to be more creative and may show leadership ability.

There is a literature that addresses giftedness as well as cultural and linguistic diversity. The identification of these youth is fraught with complexity because measures of cognitive functioning are required. Many such tests have been documented as unfair to ethnic minorities (e.g., Reynolds & Carson, 2005), including those who are economically disadvantaged and those whose first language is not English, primarily because there is a substantial language component in these tests (Bernal, 1993). Exacerbating the problem is educators' limited understanding of behaviors and characteristics indicative of giftedness in culturally and linguistically diverse youth (Kogan, 2001). Trying to evaluate individuals for giftedness is in itself a complex undertaking but the task becomes even more complex when linguistic and cultural diversity are factored in. It is also possible that what is believed to constitute giftedness varies by culture, further increasing the complexity of identifying gifted youth.

It is also possible to be gifted and learning disabled, or gifted and diagnosed as having attention-deficit hyperactivity disorder (ADHD), or a number of other possible combinations of the strength of giftedness with a weakness or limitation. Thus, giftedness is only one aspect of an individual's being and functioning. This possibility underscores the need for flexibility and uniqueness in interventions. Schoolwide enrichment models offer one means to meet the challenge of accommodating multiple and varied needs (Reis & Renzulli, 2004). Competent professional school psychologists can help to meet various needs of this population.

Physical/Health Limitations

Physical limitations include health concerns and restrictions upon an individual's personal mobility. Often when disabilities are thought of, the visible physical ones come to mind, but many health concerns are not necessarily visible to observers. Chronic health concerns, such as diabetes and asthma, as well as those that are typically finite in duration, such as a bone fracture, impact education and personal adjustment. There is no single correct manner for addressing these concerns; the supports and interventions should be specific to the child's unique needs. Some of these health concerns are low-incidence concerns that impact schooling and education in varied ways (see Phelps, 1998). Moreover, children from low-income and ethnic minority backgrounds are at significant risk for health-related difficulty (Phelps, 2005) that is often exacerbated by inadequate prenatal care (National Institute of Child Health and Human Development, 2000) and delays in obtaining federally funded early intervention services. Exposure to neurotoxins, specifically prenatal exposure to cocaine and alcohol, and high levels of lead exposure have psychoeducational manifestations. Assistance to children can come through (1) the requirements of legislation and (2) the help of professionals in the schools.

Requirements of Legislation

For some medically fragile and physically limited children to attend school, accommodations to the environment/school setting are needed. The accommodations needed vary according to the child's limitations and needs. Some environmental adjustments are now mandated as a matter of course. The Americans with Disabilities Act (ADA, 1990) requires public facilities, which include schools, to be accessible; accessibility includes access to and within the building. To meet the requirements of the law, many public schools have made needed renovations, among which were the addition of elevators and ramps, hardware that permits doors to be opened readily, and large bathroom stalls and bathroom washbasins of appropriate height. These, in fact, address only part of the need. The needs of a wheelchair-bound youngster in a mainstream classroom require considerable attention to detail that may be specific to the individual child. For example, the aisles in the classroom must be wide enough for the wheelchair to move about readily; the ideal situation is for this accommodation to occur as a matter of course, yet it will not occur without advance planning. Other details include such things as arranging materials so the wheelchair-bound child can access them independently, and when that is genuinely not practicable, making provisions for the child's comfort and needs without undue disruption of classroom routines. It is highly desirable to make accommodations in ways that do not disrupt routines as this allows for a more seamless, natural integration of the wheelchair-bound child into the mainstream classroom, which strengthens the sense of community.

Not uncommon, however, is for a child with physical limitations to have additional health-related needs. This often requires the presence and involvement of additional adults in the school environment (i.e., paraprofessionals, school nurse), to meet the child's medically related needs while ensuring appropriate instruction. Medical equipment or related procedures (e.g., catheterization) may be needed during the school day.

Children may also have other physical needs that are not visible with the naked eye. For example, a child may be diabetic. Accommodations are often required, as are specialized services, which are part of the mandated free appropriate public education. A diabetic child will need to have test supplies available and may need assistance monitoring his or her blood sugar. Other children may have dietary restrictions, or require nursing services, adaptive devices, scheduling and test accommodations, and so forth. The array of needs requiring accommodation span the continuum from time limited to ongoing; similarly, the needs and disorders range from minimal and straightforward to complex and involved (see Phelps, 1998).

Roles of Professionals in the School

School-based professionals serving in a variety of roles are essential to the success of children who have physical and/or health limitations. The advent of school-based clinician and health services may provide expanded opportunities to intervene. School psychologists are not the only individuals who can provide these services; however, their broad training in educational and developmental issues makes the professional school psychologist the individual capable of providing the most comprehensive, thorough, and integrated services. Among the possible roles of this professional are (1) child advocacy, (2) direct service provision, (3) health promotion consultation, (4) coordination of services, (5) program development and administration, and (6) applied research (Power, DuPaul, Shapiro, & Parrish, 1998).

Child advocacy includes being sufficiently knowledgeable to collaborate with others to meet the complex educational, social, interpersonal, and treatment compliance needs of the child with medical conditions (Wodrich & Pfeiffer, 1989). Training parents to be effective advocates for their child is also important. Parents often need to be better informed about (1) their child's educational, social and emotional needs, (2) the possible accommodations available, (3) working with school personnel, and (4) understanding the laws and regulations that apply to their child (Ylvisaker, Hartwick, & Stevens, 1991).

Direct service provision by school psychologists so trained can include providing behavioral interventions to manage physical/health concerns. Multiple component treatments using combinations of strategies such as positive reinforcement, practice, and self-monitoring (e.g., Steege & Harper, 1989) can be effectively applied. For example, the same combinations of behavioral strategies and interventions that can be used to manage one problem can be adapted to address another. Moreover, this is consistent with a body of research indicating that treatments that are composed of multiple components have research support (Kazdin & Weisz, 2003) for the treatment of a variety of child-adolescent problems. Children with physical/health concerns may also have related academic, behavioral, and social-emotional concerns; school psychologists intervene directly and collaborate with teachers and parents to develop plans that are effective for these students.

Schools can provide a venue to promote health (Talley & Short, 1995). Among the possibilities are (1) health education, (2) physical education, (3) health services, (4) nutrition services, (5) health promotion for staff, (6) counseling, psychological, and social services, (7) a healthy school environment, and (8) parental and community involvement. The services would be provided by appropriately trained professionals for the particular task. All services provided in the school setting should be coordinated; this limits duplication of effort and makes it more likely that a variety of needs will be addressed.

Program development and administration is an important role, providing opportunities to incorporate the most contemporary practices in programs to help children. Depending on the setting, the services might be wholly within a school, within a model in which schools are linked to other settings that provide some of the services, or to clinic settings. School psychologists can be trained for these leadership roles, but this training is generally limited to the doctoral level, as the curriculum at the specialist (certificate) level is too crowded to include this instruction. Applied research offers school psychologists an opportunity to determine the effectiveness of programs (Power et al., 1998).

Ethnic/Cultural Background

SEXUAL ORIENTATION

There is an emerging literature in school psychology on sexual minority youth (e.g., Hollander, 2000; McCabe & Rubinson, 2008; Tharinger & Wells, 2000). This literature is not limited to gay/lesbian/bisexual youth and includes those whose gender identification is atypical (Haldeman, 2000). This is long overdue considering that the one commonality shared by such youth is that all attend school. Although the main focus is obviously on the target youth, issues related to youth whose parents represent sexual diversity have also gained attention (Ryan & Martin, 2000). Moreover, the interaction of other diversity indicators, such as race, ethnicity, and religion, with sexual diversity should be considered, despite an absence of available information that is authoritative. The key point is that these individuals represent a diverse (sub)group with varied issues and concerns of their own.

Bahr, Brish, and Crouteau (2000) considered sexual minority youth within the context of the ethical code of the National Association of School Psychologists (NASP, 1997). This is useful because it utilizes an organizing framework of sensitivity and social justice within the contexts of (1) professional roles and responsibilities, (2) professional competencies, and (3) professional practices. In regard to professional roles, this includes sensitivity and respect, affirmation of sexual diversity, and not engaging or condoning discriminatory practices.

Regarding professional competencies, school psychologists must monitor and be aware of their own beliefs and not allow their limitations to compromise competent service delivery. To provide competent services, school psychologists need continuing education. Appropriate professional practices include making concern for student rights and welfare known to school personnel, using sensitive assessment and intervention practices, and applying the knowledge base of allied disciplines to improve service delivery. These notions are generally consistent with the Ethical Principles of Psychologists and Code of Conduct (American Psychological Association, 2002) and the Professional Conduct Code (NASP, 2000a).

A notable exception is in the area of professional competencies. The APA code indicates that referral is appropriate if a case is outside a psychologist's expertise or if there is a personal reason that continuing with a particular case is a conflict of interest. In contrast, the NASP code takes into account the realities of school-based practice in that school psychologists do not choose their cases. Rather, because school psychologists are required to work with those with whom they are presented and do not necessarily have the option of making a referral, a hazard of school-based practice (particularly if the school psychologist is an employee of the school system) is highlighted. A helpful addition is in the most recent revision of the APA code (APA, 2002), which now specifically names school psychologists as being required to follow the code. Flanagan, Miller, and Jacob (2005), in their analysis of the code as it applies to school psychologists, note that the specific naming of school psychologists among those who are to follow the code provides direction and a statement of professional standards that school psychologists can share with other educators (who may not have a full appreciation of the complexities of school psychology practice).

Important for school psychologists is to recognize the complexity of the developmental process for sexually diverse youth (Tharinger & Wells, 2000) that includes becoming aware of the orientation, accepting it, and being able to integrate this orientation into their self-awareness. The taboos against discussing sexual diversity, accepting it, and affirming it are formidable barriers and potential sources of upset in schools. Moreover, such youth are at high risk for a variety of untoward outcomes, such as academic failure (Elia, 1993) and psychological distress. More recently, McCabe and Rubinson (2008) provided a theory-driven framework using the theory of planned behavior (Ajden, 1985, 1991) to advocate for sexually diverse youth. Greater understanding and acceptance of such youth potentially reduces the incidence of problems for them, and when problematic situations occur, the delivery and quality of psychological services for those who require them are facilitated.

SPIRITUALITY/RELIGION

Although religion is generally absent from the school psychology literature (Halstead, 2005), it remains an important variable in understanding the thinking, attitudes, and behavior of children. Religion is particularly diverse in the United States. According to the American Religious Identification Survey (ARIS, 2008; retrieved April 30, 2009, from http://b27.cc.trincoll. edu/weblogs/AmericanReligionSurvey-ARIS/reports/ARIS_Report_2008. pdf), of the approximately 95% of adults who responded, 76% identify as Christian, approximately 4% identify as belonging to a non-Christian religion, and 15% did not identify with any religion. Approximately 5% of adults did not know which religion they belonged to or they refused to respond to the question. Christians are further subdivided into approximately one-third Catholic and two-thirds non-Catholic (comprised of numerous Protestant denominations, such as Baptist, Presbyterian, Born-Again, and so forth). Non-Christian denominations include Judaism, Islam, Buddhism, and other Eastern religions.

The effect of religion on a student's development may be positive or negative. The positive aspects include a close knit family life and greater resiliency (Overstreet & Braun, 1999); negative aspects may include less emphasis on the development of autonomy (McIntosh, D. N., & Spilka, 1998). Religion is a dimension of culture in that it identifies festivals and rites of passage, provides inspiration to achieve (Halstead, 2005), and embraces specific practices. The relationship between religion and culture is varied. The requirements, beliefs, and traditions of some religions clash with public school scheduling; there is variation in how this is addressed, although there are federal guidelines issued by the U.S. Department of Education (2003; retrieved April 20, 2009, from www.ed.gov/policy/gen/guid/religionandschools/prayer_guidance.html) on constitutionally protected prayer in public schools that outline how schools are expected to negotiate variety, respect traditions, and allow time for students to meet religious obligations without academic penalty.

Thus, religion plays a role in the life of schools and children, despite the secular nature of public education. Teaching about religion in schools has increased, the breadth of religious diversity is acknowledged in schools, and, at the same time, there has been an increase in discrimination and prejudice on religious grounds (Halstead, 2005). The agenda for school psychology (Halstead, 2005) includes professionals examining their own personal values, learning about others' values, and negotiating circumstances with sensitivity and skill. This refers to the development of cultural competence in regard to religious diversity that includes the practices, policies, attitudes, and behavior of professionals (Davis, 1997).

TWELVE

Professional Identification

The purpose of this concluding chapter is to cover the professional identification and affiliations of school psychologists. In addition there is discussion of matters highly related to professional identification including job satisfaction, the current demographic status of the specialty, and future challenges related to maintaining an adequate base of professionals in the specialty. Then we briefly describe the wide variety of professional organizations that maintain control over school psychology by setting standards for self-governance of the profession. Finally, a brief discussion of the responsibility and mechanisms for continued professional development of school psychology professionals is presented.

A Profession with Many Roles

The chapters in this book should make it clear that school psychology comprises varying levels of training for entry; diverse roles held in diverse settings; and an ever-expanding list of problems, populations, and procedures in the service of helping individuals benefit from education. Needless to say, there are several heated debates within the profession, such as best practices for assessment of learning disabilities, appropriate entry-level training into the field, and professional identification. Because of this diversity and differences of opinion, it is possible to stand two school psychologists next to each other and get two quite different perspectives on their roles. Merrell, Ervin, and Gimpel (2006) did just that by interviewing six different individuals to learn their perspective on their professional identification within school psychology. In two of the cases the school psychologists were trained at the specialist level and were working in public schools. They had relatively traditional roles including significant amounts of assessment (both normative and curriculum based) for special education eligibility and consultation regarding behavior problems. Another doctoral-level school psychologist had a strong affiliation with the local university school psychology training program and considered herself a partner in the training of future school psychologists. The next school psychologist worked in a school district in an administrative position as coordinator of research and special projects. The majority of his time was spent conducting program evaluation and effectiveness studies on the district's initiatives. The next school psychologist worked in a private, nonprofit educational organization that serves students with autism and other developmental disabilities. She spent most of her time training and consulting to help teachers learn functional behavioral assessment and running the parent education and training program. The parent programs are consistent with parents as partners as discussed in chapter 6. The final school psychologist profiled was a university professor who trained the next generation of school psychologists. Her role included teaching, research, and service, and she is afforded a significant amount of flexibility, as faculty members are not tied to the public school work schedules. Merrell and colleagues' fascinating approach to examining the current professional identity of school psychologists is worth reading in detail. The authors note that an important trend in the interviews was that each school psychologist's role appeared to develop and change over time, but that they are all tied together by the desire to help individuals benefit from their educational experiences.

Dual Professional Identity

At the most basic level, school psychologists identify themselves as professionals. A profession has several characteristics (see sidebar). School psychology under the auspices of APA and NASP meet these criteria for being a profession and, therefore, the claim that school psychology is a profession is valid. The challenge comes when we try to clarify whether school psychology's identity is with professional psychology or education.

As discussed in chapter 1, school psychology is regulated by professional psychology credentialing procedures in association with the American Psychological Association and state boards of psychology for licensure of psychologists and by education credentialing procedures in association with the National Association of School Psychologists (NASP) and state boards of education credentialing processes. Thus, Tharinger, Pryzwansky, and Miller (2008) suggest that school psychology has a dual professional identity stemming from the two professional homes (APA and NASP) of the specialty. These dual professional homes are about more than level of training (doctoral versus subdoctoral). Rather, they are about the affiliation with the professions of either psychology or education. In either case, there is substantial cross affiliation, as school psychologists are both psychologists and partners in education. The distinction is a matter of degree. That is, the school psychologist's identity may be primarily with psychology and tangentially with education. On the other hand, identification may reside with education primarily and partially with psychology. This is consistent with the role NASP plays in credentialing training programs in which NASP is the

A profession requires

1. Mastery of a complex body of knowledge and skills that are used in the service of others

2. A system of accountability to the public for minimum standards of competence and ethics

3. Autonomy in practice and judgment

4. Self-regulation through certification, licensure, and accreditation

(Cruess, Johnston, & Cruess, 2004; Rice & Duncan, 2006)

specialized professional agency (SPA) that nationally recognizes programs for the National Council for Accreditation of Teacher Education (NCATE). Other SPAs in NCATE nationally recognize training programs in mathematics, reading, early childhood, and educational leadership. Certainly there are exceptions to the principle of dual professional identity, but in most cases this is the situation.

Therefore, there are some school psychologists whose professional identity is strongly tied to professional psychology—and they would say, "I am a psychologist in the schools." There are some whose professional identity is more strongly tied to education—and they would say, "I am a school psychologist." Although there appear to be two dominant professional identities for professional psychologists, it could be argued that there is a third. That is, there are others whose identity is defined by their workplace, —for example, to help children to learn at such-and-such school district—and they would say, "I am a school psychologist at *Wonderful* School District." These individuals exhibit a strong affinity for their school or school district and are likely not inclined to join professional organizations espousing either psychology or education as the emphasis of the identity of school psychology.

Although a dual identity causes some conflicts within the profession, it has also made for a rich partnership. School psychology, from the perspective of NASP and specialist level training, has benefited from the connection with APA and the broader field of professional psychology. This has allowed school psychologists to practice in a variety of settings and expand their role, such as including neuropsychology and psychotherapy among their competencies. As well, doctoral-level school psychology has benefited from the strong connection with schools and from maintaining the central role school psychologists play in the formal education of children.

Profile of Current School Psychologists

A number of studies have examined the demographic characteristics of practicing school psychologists. Curtis, Hunley, and Grier (2004) summarized the findings from several of these studies. Based on their data, school psychologists are predominantly Caucasian (93%). Approximately 70% of practicing school psychologists are female and as many as 80% of students in school psychology training programs are female. School psychologists tend to be trained at the specialist level. About 97% were trained at the specialist level or above; and Curtis and colleagues note that only 16% of these individuals were trained at the doctoral level, suggesting that this trend of predominantly specialist-level training will continue. With regard to age, the mean age of practicing school psychologists and university trainers was in the mid-40s with university trainers being slightly older and having more years of experience. Fagan (2004) cautions that with the aging of Americans in the baby-boom generation, school psychology could face more shortages than it is currently experiencing. School psychologists work primarily in public schools (77.5%) with only 6.3% working in university settings. As can be seen in most of these demographics, school psychologists are not representative of the diversity of the United States. This raises concerns about the ability of the specialty to meet the needs of diverse populations as well as to attract members of these populations to its ranks (Davis, McIntosh, Phelps, & Kehle, 2004).

Job Satisfaction

Reschly and Wilson (1995) surveyed school psychologists in 1986 and 1991–1992 to determine trends in job satisfaction. They looked at job satisfaction for university faculty and practicing professionals. Results indicated that faculty members had higher levels of job satisfaction, but that overall both groups reported positive job satisfaction. For the practitioners, job dissatisfaction was associated with a lack of career advancement opportunities. In a comparison of school psychologists that serve a single school versus those that serve multiple schools, Proctor and Steadman (2003) again found that overall school psychologists reported high job satisfaction, but school psychologists who served only a single school reported higher job satisfaction and lower feeling of burnout than those serving multiple schools. Using meta-analysis, VanVoorhis and Levinson (2006) found that nearly 85% of 2,116 school psychologists were at least satisfied with their job.

School Psychology Personnel Shortage

These data on the stability of job satisfaction for school psychologists over the years seem to be in sharp contrast to the shortage of both school psychology practitioners and trainers. Relevant to the identity of the school psychologist are issues that may account for the shortage in their ranks; personnel shortages are a reality the specialty of school psychology must address, as other areas of professional psychology are not experiencing similar shortages (McIntosh, D. E., 2004). Further, there has been a shortage of school psychologists for many years—in fact, for decades—historically because of the rapid expansion of the specialty (Fagan, 2004). School psychology is currently facing a shortage of both trainers and practitioners for a number of reasons. First, school psychologists are not always understood as affiliated with professional psychology; rather, they are associated with school counselors or guidance counselors (Davis, A. S., et al., 2004). Consequently, individuals interested in professional psychology as a career do not realize that school psychology is an option (Graves & Wright, 2007; Merrell et al., 2006). Another possible reason for the shortage is that school psychologists spend a majority of their time conducting assessments for special education placement decisions when they would prefer to be engaged in prevention and consultative activities (Hosp & Reschly, 2002). Indeed, this knowledge could discourage potential school psychology students who would prefer broader practice. Also, as previously discussed, the lack of diversity in school psychology may deter individuals who are not Caucasian from considering the profession as a career option. Regardless of the cause, an ongoing shortage of school psychologists will likely result in the responsibilities being taken up by other mental health service providers. Crespi and Politikos (2004) note that there is a surplus of clinical psychologists and because of the surplus they are experiencing decreases in salary and increased competition. It is reasonable to assume that clinical psychologists among others will be seeking entry into positions not filled because of the school psychology shortage. Along these same lines, because school psychology has the tradition of including subdoctoral entry into the field, the void will likely be filled by the vast number of practitioners with subdoctoral mental health credentials. Graves and Wright (2007) summarized various researchers' views on the potential impact of continued shortages of school psychologists: "(a) higher ratios of school psychologists to students, (b) more time in special education eligibility activities with less time in intervention-based services, (c) lower standards for credentialing, and (d) larger enrollments in training programs, but with fewer faculty" (p. 865). As Crespi and Politikos note, school psychology is facing a "looming crisis" (2004, p. 473).

Why Become a School Psychologist?

Given the shortage of school psychologists in both practice and academe, it is important to ask, "Why become a school psychologist?" The specialty of school psychology is an active, vibrant, and robust specialty in professional psychology. Further, it is a changing field, and the changes appear to be for the better. The identity of school psychology will develop as new waves of school psychologists enter the fields of practice and training. Knowing their motivations may help communicate the benefits and opportunities in school psychology as well as help show where the specialty may be headed next.

Graves and Wright (2007) asked "Why school psychology?" to over 300 current graduate students in school psychology attending programs leading to specialist, PsyD, and PhD degrees. About 65% of the respondents were in subdoctoral programs and about 75% came from undergraduate majors in psychology. This is a notable trend in which the next generation of school psychologists may increasingly identify primarily with psychology as a professional identity. As for postgraduate employment, about 86% planned to work in a public school setting. The only differences between doctoral and subdoctoral motivations for pursuing school psychology were job stability and public school work schedule, which were more important to the students seeking subdoctoral credentials. For both groups the highest rated motivations were a desire to work with children, working in a school environment, job stability, and public school work schedule. Graves and Wright also asked open-ended questions about additional factors that lead to an interest in school psychology and again found *interest in working with children* as a primary reason. However, the most frequent reason was *personal experiences with school psychologists* in the course of schooling and other settings. Consistent with our graduate students reports, the personal experiences described by Graves and Wright mentioned respondents having seen the school psychologists in their personal experience not do as much as they could have, and expression of a desire by the respondents to make the field better. Although personal experiences influenced only 30% of the sample, these reports may be an indication that school psychologists need to broaden their role so as to have maximal impact on the lives of students in the schools where they serve.

With regard to becoming a university trainer in school psychology, Nagle, Suldo, Christenson, and Hansen (2004) conducted focus groups and surveyed over 200 current graduate students in school psychology to determine the reasons they would be interested in a position in academe. Of the graduate students interested in academe, the role of academics such as working with students, flexibility, and stimulating work environment were the highest ranked reasons. Interestingly, salary and status were not major factors in their deciding to seek a position in academe. The major deterrent to a role in academe was job stress. Respondents suggested ways to make a career in academe more inviting including increased salary, more opportunities for applied work, and decreased politics.

Professional Organizations in School Psychology

In part because of the dual identity of school psychology, the specialty is represented by more than one professional organization. Tharinger, Pryzwansky, and Miller (2008) provided a brief overview of these organizations and the following is adopted from that work.

APA DIVISION 16 (SCHOOL PSYCHOLOGY)

The Division of School Psychology (Division 16) within APA is one of 54 divisions of the APA, represents doctoral school psychology, and has approximately 2,000 members. APA is the largest organization representing psychologists in the United States, representing over 150,000 psychologists and associates. Division 16 is a highly organized group within the infrastructure of APA and is charged with representing scientist-practitioner psychologists whose research and practice interests have to do with children, families, and schooling. The division is interested in promoting high-quality education and training of psychologists and school psychologists, increasing effective and collaborative psychological practice in schools, supporting ethical and socially responsible practices, and encouraging scholarly publications in school psychology. The division publishes the APA journal *School Psychology Quarterly* as well as the quarterly newsletter *The School Psychologist*. Through representation on

---

School Psychology Organizations
- American Psychological Association (APA) Division 16 (School Psychology)
- National Association of School Psychologists (NASP)
- Council of Directors of School Psychology Training Programs (CDSPP)
- Trainers of School Psychologists (TSP)
- Society for the Study of School Psychology (SSSP)
- American Board of School Psychology (ABSP)
- American Academy of School Psychology (AASP)
- International School Psychology Association (ISPA)
- School Psychology Specialty Council (SPSC)

---

the Ethics Code Task Force, Division 16 contributes to the development and revisions of the APA Ethics Code. Division 16 is involved in training program accreditation through representation on the APA Commission on Accreditation. Division 16 sponsors the activities of the graduate student organization for school psychologists named Student Affiliates in School Psychology. The division also annually recognizes distinction through its Senior Scientist, Bardon Distinguished Service, Witmer Early Career, Outstanding Dissertation, and the Henkin Student Travel awards.

NATIONAL ASSOCIATION OF SCHOOL PSYCHOLOGISTS

NASP is the largest national organization serving exclusively the interests of school psychologists and reportedly has approximately 22,000 members comprised of school psychologists, trainers, and students. NASP was founded in 1969 and has a focus on advocacy for children's needs; it represents both specialist and doctoral school psychology practitioners and educators and trainers in specialist and doctoral programs. Although NASP was originally founded to represent primarily nondoctoral school psychology practitioners and their trainers, NASP successfully developed a professional template to represent both nondoctoral and doctoral members of the field. NASP has developed *Standards for Training and Field Placements for Programs in School Psychology* (2000b); *Standards for the Credentialing of School Psychologists* (2000); a *Professional Conduct Manual* (2000a), which includes *Principles for Professional Ethics* (2000) and *Guidelines for the Provision of School Psychological Services*; and the third edition of *School Psychology: A Blueprint for Training and Practice* (III) (2006). Further, NASP approves training programs and grants an entry-level credential, the Nationally Certified School Psychologist (NCSP). In addition, NASP publishes a journal, *School Psychology Review* and a newsletter, *Communiqué,* and has a website at www.nasponline.org. NASP also offers many books and products through NASP Publications and holds an annual convention.

COUNCIL OF DIRECTORS OF SCHOOL PSYCHOLOGY TRAINING PROGRAMS

The Council of Directors of School Psychology Training Programs (CDSPP) is comprised of programs from North American doctoral training programs in school psychology. Membership is at the training program level with each program having one vote. Program representation is provided through the program director, but all program faculty are encouraged to participate in professional activities such as the annual meetings. Accreditation by APA is not required for membership, although attending to accreditation issues is of primary interest in CDSPP's leadership of the field.

TRAINERS OF SCHOOL PSYCHOLOGISTS

Similar to CDSPP, Trainers of School Psychologists (TSP) is comprised of both specialist and doctoral training programs as institutional members. TSP provides collaborative networks among trainers through sponsoring trainers' workshops held during the NASP annual convention. In addition, TSP publishes a quarterly newsletter entitled *Trainers' Forum*. TSP maintains a website that, among other things, announces the winner of the Outstanding Contributions to Training Annual Award. TSP also provides small scholarship grants to junior faculty and graduate students.

SOCIETY FOR THE STUDY OF SCHOOL PSYCHOLOGY

The Society for the Study of School Psychology (SSSP) is devoted exclusively to promoting, recognizing, and disseminating scholarship and research in school psychology, as well as promoting the profession of school psychology. SSSP evolved from the group that established the *Journal of School Psychology* (*JSP*). The conversion to a not-for-profit society enabled SSSP to distribute resources to benefit the profession, including maintaining operational responsibility for their prestigious journal. SSSP provides research grants and sponsors a biannual conference to connect junior faculty with senior researchers. The current membership consists of members from the original JSP corporation and members elected to society membership.

AMERICAN BOARD OF SCHOOL PSYCHOLOGY

The American Board of School Psychology recognizes professional psychologists in the specialty of school psychology through a board certification evaluation process. Available to psychologists licensed by their state board of psychology, the process for becoming board certified requires an education and training review, work samples, and a face-to-face examination that covers the work samples, ethics, research, and practice issues. This voluntary competency-based credential is governed by the American Board of Professional Psychology (ABPP), which also oversees 12 other psychology specialties. Board certification in school psychology has been available since 1968.

AMERICAN ACADEMY OF SCHOOL PSYCHOLOGY

The American Academy of School Psychology (AASP) is comprised of all psychologists who are board certified in school psychology by the ABPP. The AASP is dedicated to the application of the science and profession of psychology to issues related to the protection and promotion of children and youth. The AASP provides an opportunity for its members to work closely with other fellows on the promotion of the specialty practice of school psychology at its highest level.

INTERNATIONAL SCHOOL PSYCHOLOGY ASSOCIATION

The International School Psychology Association (ISPA) is an organization of psychologists working to promote the spread of school psychology, particularly in countries where school psychology is not fully established. ISPA is recognized by the United Nations as an important nongovernmental organization. Membership is open to individual school psychologists and graduate students. There are ISPA affiliates or ISPA mission partners for organizations around the world that share a similar mission. ISPA publishes a newsletter entitled *World*Go*Round* and a scholarly journal, *School Psychology International*. In addition, ISPA has produced a code of ethics and international guidelines for the preparation of school psychologists.

SCHOOL PSYCHOLOGY SPECIALTY COUNCIL

The School Psychology Specialty Council (SPSC), originally known as the School Psychology Synarchy, was established as a forum to allow the major school psychology organizations to coordinate and collaborate on cross-cutting tasks important to education, training, and maintaining the specialty in school psychology. Members include the school psychology organizations described above. In addition to promoting communication among the members, the SPSC holds a seat on the board of directors of the Council of Specialties (for more information see http://cospp.org) that facilitates interaction between the specialty of school psychology and 11 other specialties in professional psychology.

Professional Development and Continuing Education

It seems fitting to end this book on the topic of continuing education because a central commitment of school psychologists is to lifelong learning. Consonant with a theme in this book, school psychology is an evolving profession that will continue to evolve well past the publication date of this book, and it will do so in large part because of the professional development each school psychologist has committed to as part of his or her professional identity. It is apparent to school psychology professionals that their training is insufficient to maintain the level of knowledge to practice competently over their careers (Fagan, 2000). The fields of psychology and education are perpetually evolving in terms of development of new practice standards, development of new knowledge such as the explosion of information from neuroscience, changes in federal and state laws, and updates to ethics codes of practices.

The need to remain current with the specialty of school psychology has been formally recognized by both major professional organizations in school psychology. For APA, the responsibility to maintain competence is in the APA *Ethical Principles of Psychologists and Code of Conduct* (2002). Similarly, the responsibility for continuing professional development is codified by NASP in the *Professional Conduct Manual* (2000). In terms of credentials, NASP offers the Nationally Certified School Psychologists (NCSP) credential which graduates of NASP-accredited school psychology programs are eligible to earn. Maintaining the credential requires 75 hours of continuing professional development every 3 years. Similarly, school psychologists licensed by their state board of psychology have continuing education requirements to maintain their license. Every state is different, but there are typically 2- or 3-year cycles of licensure renewal that require evidence of continuing education. Many states require continuing education specific to ethics as well. National and local professional organizations provide substantial opportunities to practicing school psychologists to gain continuing professional development credits. The APA authorizes a variety of providers of APA-approved continuing education credits such as state psychological associations and other professional groups. The national conventions of both APA and NASP provide many opportunities through workshops designated as qualifying for continuing education. For trainers, teaching courses and writing scholarly articles typically qualify for continuing education credits. Finally, book study, audio programs, and now Internet-based programs are increasingly popular for school psychologists in meeting their continuing education needs associated with ever-expanding roles and responsibilities.

REFERENCES

Achenbach, T. M., & Rescorla, L. A. (2001). *Manual for ASEBA school age forms and profiles*. Burlington, VT: University of Burlington Center for Children, Youth and Families.

Achenbach, T. M., & Rescorla, L. (2003). *The Achenbach System of Empirically Based assessment*. Burlington: University of Vermont.

Ajden, I. (1985). From intentions to actions: A theory of planned behavior. In J. Kuhland & J. Beckman (Eds.), *Action–control: From cognition to behavior* (pp. 11–38). Heidelberg: Springer.

Adjen, I. (1991). A theory of planned behavior. *Organizational Behavior and Human Decision Processes, 50,* 179–211.

Allen, I. E., & Seaman, J. (2008). Staying the course— Online education in the United States, 2008. Available at ww.sloanc.org/publications/survey/pdf/staying_the_course.pdf.

Alvord, M. K., & Grados, J. J. (2005). Enhancing resilience in children: A proactive approach. *Professional Psychology: Research and Practice, 36*(3), 238–245.

American Board of School Psychology. (2007). *Examiner's manual for board certification in school psychology*. Savannah, GA: Author.

American Counseling Association (ACA). (1997). *Definition of professional counseling*. Retrieved July 24, 2008, from www.aca.org.

American Educational Research Association, American Psychological Association, & National Council on Measurement in Education. (1999). *Standards for educational and psychological testing*. Washington, DC: American Educational Research Association.

American Psychiatric Association. (2000). *Diagnostic and statistical manual of mental disorders* (4th ed., text revision). Washington, DC: Author.

American Psychological Association (APA). (1981). Specialty guidelines for the provision of services by school psychologists. *American Psychologist, 36,* 670–681.

American Psychological Association (APA). (1992). *Ethical principles of psychologists and code of conduct*. Washington, DC: Author.

American Psychological Association (APA). (2002). Ethical principles of psychologists and code of conduct. *American Psychologist, 57,* 1060–1073.

American Psychological Association (APA). (2005). *Archival description of school psychology specialty*. Washington, DC: Author. Retrieved July 10, 2007, from *www.apa.org/crsppp/schpsych.html.*

American Religious Identification Survey (2008). Retrieved April 30, 2009, from http://b27.cc.trincoll.edu/Weblogs/AmericanReligionSurvey- ARIS/reports/ARIS Report 2008.pdf.

Americans with Disabilities Act of 1990 or ADA. Pub.L. No. 101-136), 42 U.S.C. § 12101. Regulations appear at 28 C.F.R. Part 35 (1996).

Anastasi, A. (1988). *Psychological testing* (6th ed.). New York: Macmillan.

Anderson, J. R. (2004). *Cognitive psychology and its implications* (6th ed.). New York: Worth.

Ardoin, S. P. (2006). The response in response to intervention: Evaluating the utility of assessing maintenance of intervention effects. *Psychology in the Schools, 43*(6), 713–725.

Ardoin, S. P., & Christ, T. J. (2008). Evaluating curriculum-based measurement slope estimates using data from triannual universal screenings. *School Psychology Review, 37*, 109–125.

Aten, J. D., Strain, J. D., & Gillespie, R. E. (2008). A transtheoretical model of supervision. *Training and Education in Professional Psychology, 2*, 1–9.

August, D., & Hakuta, K. (1998). *Educating language-minority children.* Washington, DC: National Academy Press.

Babinski, L. M., Knotek, S. E., & Rogers, D. L. (2004). Facilitating conceptual change. in new teacher consultation groups. In N. M. Lambert, I. Hylander, & J. H. Sandoval (Eds.), *Consultee-centered consultation* (pp. 101–113). Mahwah, NJ: Erlbaum.

Baca, L. M. (1998). Bilingualism and bilingual education. In L. M. Baca & H. Cervantes (Eds.), *The bilingual special education interface* (3rd ed., pp. 26–45). Columbus, OH: Merrill.

Baddeley, A. (2003). Working memory: Looking back and looking forward. *Nature Reviews Neuroscience, 4*, 829-839.

Bahr, M. W., Brish, B., & Crouteau, J. M. (2000). Addressing sexual orientation and professional ethics in the training of school psychologists in school and university settings. *School Psychology Review, 29*, 217–230.

Bandura, A. (1978). The self system in reciprocal determinism. *American Psychologist, 33*(4), 344–358.

Baker, C. (2001). *Foundations of bilingual education and bilingualism.* Clevedon, U.K.: Multilingual Matters.

Barber, J. P., Sharpless, B. A., Klostermann, S., & McCarthy, K. S. (2007). Assessing intervention competence and its relation to therapy outcome: A selected review derived from the outcome literature. *Professional Psychology: Research and Practice. 38*, 493–500.

Barkley, R. A. (1997). *ADHD and the nature of self-control.* New York: Guilford Press.

Barnett, J. E., Doll, B., Younggren, J. N., & Rubin, N. J. (2007). Clinical competence for practicing psychologists: Clearly a work in progress. *Professional Psychology: Research and Practice, 38*, 510–517.

Barrett, P. M., & Short, A. L. (2003). Parental involvement in the treatment of anxious children. In A. E. Kazdin, & J. R. Weisz, (Eds.), *Evidence-based psychotherapies for children and adolescents* (pp. 101–119). New York: Guilford Press.

Barton, A. C., Drake, C., Perez, J. G., St. Louis, K., & George, M. (2004). Ecologies of parental engagement in urban education. *Educational Researcher, 33*, 3–12.

Bassan-Diamond, L. E., Teglasi, H., & Schmitt, P. (1995).Temperament and a story-telling measure of self-regulation. *Journal of Research in Personality, 29*, 109–120.

Batsche, G. M., Castillo, J. M., Dixon, D. N., & Forde, S. (2008). Best practices in linking assessment to intervention. In A. Thomas & J. Grimes (Eds.), *Best practices in school psychology* (5th ed., pp 177–194). Bethesda, MD: National Association of School Psychologists.

Beck, A. T., & Emery, G. (1985). *Anxiety disorders and phobias: A cognitive perspective.* New York: Basic Books.

Bergan, J. (1977). *Behavioral consultation.* Columbus. OH: Merrill.

Bergan, J. R., & Kratochwill, T. R. (1990). *Behavioral consultation.* New York : Plenum Press.

Bergan, J. R., & Schnaps, A. (1983). A model for instructional consultation. In J. Alpert & J. Meyers (Eds.), *Training in consultation* (pp. 104–119). Springfield, IL: Thomas.

Bernal, M. (1993). *Ethnic identity: Formation and transmission among Hispanics and other minorities.* Albany, NY: State University of New York Press.

Bernard, M. E., Ellis, A., & Terjesen, M. D. (2006). Rational-emotive behavioral approaches to childhood disorders: History, theory, practice and research. In A. Ellis & M. E. Bernard (Eds.), *Rational emotive behavioral approaches to childhood disorders: Theory, practice and research* (pp. 3–84). New York: Springer.

Bernard, M. E., & Joyce, M. (1984). *Rational –emotive therapy with children and adolescents: Theory, treatment strategies, and preventative methods.* New York: Wiley.

Bersoff, D. N. (1994). Ethical ambiguity: The 1992 ethics code as oxymoron. *Professional Psychology: Research and Practice, 25,* 382–387.

Blankman, C., Teglasi, H. , & Lawser, M. (2002). Thematic apperception, narrative schemas, and literacy. *Journal of Psychoeducational Assessment, 20,* 268–289.

Bolman, L. G., & Deal, T. E. (2003). *Reframing organizations: Artistry, choice, and leadership* (3rd ed.). San Francisco, CA: Jossey-Bass.

Bordin, E. S. (1994). Theory and research on the therapeutic alliance: New directions. In A. O. Horvath & L. S. Greenberg (Eds.), *The working alliance: Theory, research and practice* (pp. 13–37). Oxford, England: Wiley.

Bracken, B. A., Keith, L. K., & Walker, K. C. (1998). Assessment of preschool behavior and social-emotional functioning: A review of thirteen third-party instruments. *Journal of Psychoeducational Assessment, 26,* 155–166.

Bracken, B. A., & McCallum, R. S. (1998). *Universal Nonverbal Intelligence Test.* Itasca, IL: Riverside.

Braden, J., DiMarino-Linnen, E., & Good, T. L. (2001). Schools, society and school psychologists: History and future directions. *Journal of School Psychology, 39,* 203–219.

Braden, M. D., & Miller, J. A. (2007). Increasing parental involvement in education. *Communiqué, 36*(1), 39–42.

Brammer, L. M., Shostrum E. L., & Abrego, P. J. (1989). *Therapeutic psychology: Fundamentals of counseling and psychotherapy* (5th ed.). Englewood Cliffs, NJ: Prentice-Hall.

Brodin, M. (2004). What does he look like? In N. M. Lambert, I. Hylander, & J. H. Sandoval (Eds.), *Consultee-centered consultation* (pp. 265–278). Mahwah, NJ: Erlbaum.

Bronfenbrenner, U. (1979). *The ecology of human development: Experiments by nature and design.* Cambridge, MA: Harvard University Press.

Brown, D., Pryzwansky, W. B., & Schulte, A. (1998). *Psychological consultation: An introduction to theory and practice* (4th ed.). Boston, MA: Allyn & Bacon.

Buerkle, K., Whitehouse, E. M., & Christenson, S. L. (2009). Partnering with families for educational success. In T. B. Gutkin & C. R. Reynolds (Eds.), *The handbook of school psychology* (4th ed., pp. 655–680). New York: John Wiley.

Burns, M. K., VanDerHeyden, A. M., & Boice, C. H. (2008). Best practices in delivery of intensive academic interventions. In A. Thomas & J. Grimes (Eds.), *Best practices in school psychology V* (Vol. 4, pp. 1151–1162). Bethesda, MD: National Association of School Psychologists.

Carroll, J. B. (1993). *Human cognitive abilities: A survey of factor analytic studies.* New York: Cambridge University Press.

Caplan, G. (1970). *Types of mental health consultation.* New York: Basic Books.

Caplan, G. (1995). Types of mental health consultation. *Journal of Educational and Psychological Consultation, 6,* 7–21.

Caplan, G., & Caplan, R. (1993). *Theory and practice of mental health consultation* (2nd ed.). San Francisco: Jossey-Bass.

Caplan, G., Caplan, R., & Erchul W. P. (1995). A contemporary view of mental health consultation: Comments on "Types of mental health consultation" by Gerald Caplan,1963). *Journal of Educational and Psychological Consultation, 4,* 105–112.

Cattell, R. B. (1941). Some theoretical issues in adult intelligence testing. *Psychological Bulletin, 38,* 592.

Chafouleas, S. M., Briesch, A. M., Riley-Tillman, T. C., & McCoach, D. B. (2009). Moving beyond assessment of treatment acceptability: An examination of the factor structure of the Usage Rating Profile Intervention (URP-I). *School Psychology Quarterly, 24*(1), 36–47.

Chafouleas, S. M., Clonan, S. M., & Vanauken, T. L. (2002). A national survey of current supervision and evaluation practices of school psychologists. *Psychology in the Schools, 39,* 317–325.

Christ, T. J. (2008). Best practices in problem analysis. In A. Thomas, & J. Grimes (Eds.), *Best practices in school psychology* (5th ed., pp 159–176). Bethesda, MD: National Association of School Psychologists.

Christensen, C., Johnson, C. W., & Horn, M. B. (2008). *Disrupting class: How disruptive innovation will change the way the world learns.* New York: McGraw-Hill.

Christenson, S. L. (1995). Families and schools: What is the role of the school psychologist? *School Psychology Quarterly, 10*(2), 118–132.

Clarke, G. N. (1995). Improving the transition from basic efficacy research to effectiveness studies: Methodological issues and procedures. *Journal of Consulting and Clinical Psychology, 63*(5), 718–725.

Cloud, N. (2007). Bilingual education practices. In G. B. Esquivel, E. C. Lopez., & S. Nahari (Eds.), *Handbook of multicultural school psychology* (pp. 201–221). Mahwah, NJ: Erlbaum.

Cloud, N., Genesee, F ., & Hamayan, E. (2000). *Dual-language instruction: A handbook for enriched education.* Boston: Heinle & Heinle.

Cobern, W. W. (1993). Constructivism. *Journal of Educational and Psychological Consultation, 4,* 105–112.

Cohen, R. J., & Swerdlik, M. E. (2005). *Psychological testing* (6th ed.). New York: McGraw-Hill.

Coleman, M., & Churchill, S. (1997). Challenges to family involvement. *Childhood Education, 73,* 144–148.

Cone, J. (1978). The behavior assessment grid (BAG): A conceptual framework and a taxonomy. *Behavior Therapy, 9,* 882–888.

Cone, J. (1981). Psychometric considerations. In M. Hersen, & A. Bellack, (Eds.), *Behavioral assessment: A practical handbook* (pp. 38–70). Elmsford, NY: Pergamon Press.

Conners, C. K. (2007). *Conners Behavior Rating Scales.* North Tonawanda, NY: Multi-Health Systems.

Connolly, A. J. (2007). *KeyMath-3: Diagnostic assessment.* Bloomington, MN: Pearson.

Cormier, S., & Cormier, B. (1998). *Interviewing strategies for helpers: Fundamental skills and cognitive-behavioral interventions,*(4th ed.). Belmont, CA: Thomson/Brooks Cole Publishing.

Cormier, S., & Nurius, P. (2003). *Interviewing strategies for helpers* (5th ed.). Pacific Grove, CA: Brooks-Cole.

Corsini, R. J. (1989). Introduction. In R. J. Corsini, & D. Wedding (Eds.), *Current psychother-apies* (4th ed., pp 1–16.) Itasca, IL: Peacock Press.

Corsini, R. J. (2000). Introduction. In R. J. Corsini, & D. Wedding (Eds.). *Current psychother-apies* (6th ed., pp. 1–15). Itasca, IL: Peacock Press.

Costantino, G., & Malgady, R. G. (2003). Narrative therapy for Hispanic children and adoles-cents In A. E. Kazdin, & J. R. Weisz (Eds.), *Evidence-based psychotherapies for children and adolescents* (pp. 425–438). New York: Guilford Press.

Costantino, G., Malgady, R. G., & Rogler, L. H. (1988). *TEMAS*. Los Angeles, CA: Western Psychological Services.

Cox, D. D. (2005). Evidence-based interventions using home-school collaboration. *School Psychology Quarterly, 20*(4), 473–497.

Crespi, T. D., & Politikos, N. N. (2004). Respecialization as a school psychologist: Education, training, and supervision for school practice. *Psychology in the Schools, 41*(4), 473–480.

Cronbach, L. J. (1957). The two disciplines of scientific psychology. *American Psychologist, 12,* 671–684.

Cruess, S. R., Johnston, S., & Cruess, R. L. (2004). "Profession": A working definition for med-ical educators. *Teaching and Learning in Medicine, 16*(1), 74–76.

Cummins, J. (1984). *Bilingual special education issues in assessment and pedagogy*. San Diego, CA: College Hill.

Cummins, J. (1986). Empowering minority students: A framework for interaction. *Harvard Educational Review, 56,* 18–36.

Curtis, M. J., Hunley, S. A., & Grier, E. C. (2004). The status of school psychology: Implica-tions of a major personnel shortage. *Psychology in the Schools, 41*(4), 431–442.

Curtis, M. J., Lopez, A. D., Batsche, G. M., & Smith, J. C. (2006, March). *School psychology 2005: A national perspective*. Paper presented at the National Association of School Psy-chologists, Anaheim, CA.

D'Amato, R. C., Fletcher-Janzen, E., & Reynolds, C. R. (2005). *Handbook of school neuropsy-chology*. John Wiley & Sons: Hoboken, NJ.

Dana, R. H. (2007). Culturally competent school assessment: Performance measures of per-sonality. *Psychology in the Schools, 44,* 229–242.

Darch, C., Miao, Y., & Shippen, P. (2004). A model for involving parents of children with learning and behavior problems in the schools. *Preventing School Failure, 48,* 224–34.

Davis, A. S., McIntosh, D. E., Phelps, L., & Kehle, T. J. (2004). Addressing the shortage of school psychologists: A summative overview. *Psychology in the Schools, 41*(4), 489–495.

Davis, K. (1997). *Exploring the intersection between cultural competency and managed health care policy: Implications for state and county mental health agencies*. Alexandria, VA: National Technical Assistance Center for State Mental Health Planning. Available at www.nasmhpd.org/search_action_docs.cfm.

Dean, R. S., & Woodcock, R. W. (2003). *Dean-Woodcock Neuropsychological Battery*. Itasca, IL: Riverside.

Delis, D. C., Kaplin, E., & Kramer, J. H. (2001). *Delis-Kaplin Executive Function System: Tech-nical manual*. San Antonio, TX: Psychological Corporation.

Denton, C. A., Fletcher, J. M., Anthony, J. L., & Francis, D. J. (2006). An evaluation of inten-sive intervention for students with persistent reading difficulties. *Journal of Learning Dis-abilities, 39*(5), 447–466.

Deno, S. L. (1987). Curriculum-based measurement. *Teaching Exceptional Children, 20,* 41.

Deno, S. L. (1995). School psychologist as problem solver. In A. Thomas & J. Grimes (Eds.), *Best practices in school psychology III* (pp. 471–484). Washington, DC: National Association of School Psychologists.

Di Giuseppe, R. (1990). Rational-emotive assessment of school-aged children. *School Psychology Review, 19,* 287–293.

Di Giuseppe, R. (1991). A RET model of assessment. In M. E. Bernard (Ed.), *Using rational emotive therapy effectively* (pp. 151–172). New York: Plenum Press.

Di Giuseppe, R., & Bernard. M. E. (1990). The application of rational-emotive theory and therapy to school-aged children. *School Psychology Review, 19,* 268-286.

Di Giuseppe, R., Linscott, J., & Jilton, R. (1995). Developing the therapeutic alliance in child-adolescent psychotherapy. *Applied and Preventive Psychology, 5,* 85–100.

Doll, B., LeClair, C., & Kurien, S. (2009). Effective classrooms: Classroom learning environments that foster school success. In T. B. Gutkin & C. R. Reynolds (Eds.), *The handbook of school psychology* (4th ed., pp. 791–807). New York: John Wiley.

Domitrovich, C. E., Cortes, R. C., & Greenberg, M. T. (2007). Improving young children's social and emotional competence: A randomized trial of the preschool "PATHS" curriculum. *Journal of Primary Prevention, 28*(2), 67–91.

Dretzke, J., Davenport, C., Frew, E., Stewart-Brown S., Taylor, R. S., Hyde, C., et al. (2009). The clinical effectiveness of different parenting programmes for children with conduct problems: A systematic review of randomised controlled trials. *Child and Adolescent Psychiatry and Mental Health, 3.* Retrieved July 2, 2009, from www.capmh.com/content/3/1/7.

Drewes, A. (2002). Play-based interventions are needed more now than ever. *School Psychologist, 56,* 16–18.

Duncan, B. B. (2004). School psychologists as consultee-centered consultants within a system of case framework: Service delivery and training challenges. In N. M. Lambert, Hylander, I. & J. H. Sandoval. (Eds.), *Consultee-centered consultation* (pp. 79–100). Mahwah, NJ: Erlbaum.

Eddy, J. M., Reid, J. B., & Curry, V. (2002). The etiology of youth antisocial behavior, delinquency, and violence and a public health approach to prevention. In M. R. Shinn, H. M. Walker, & G. Stoner (Eds.), *Interventions for academic and behavior problems II: Preventive and remedial approaches* (pp. 27–51). Bethesda, MD: National Association of School Psychologists.

Eddy, J. M., Reid, J. B., Stoolmiller, M., & Fetrow, R. A. (2003). Outcomes during middle school for an elementary school-based preventive intervention for conduct problems: Follow-up results from a randomized trial. *Behavior Therapy, 34*(4), 535–552.

Education for All Handicapped Children Act of 1975. Pub. L. 94–142.

Elbow, P. (1998). *Writing without teachers* (2nd ed.). New York: Oxford University Press.

Elia, J. P. (1993). Homophobia in the high school: A problem in need of a resolution. *High School Journal, 77,* 177–185.

Elliott, S. N., & Gresham, F. M. (2008). *The Social Skills Intervention System.* Minneapolis, MN: Pearson.

Elliott, S. N., Witt, J. C., Kratochwill, T. R., Stoiber, K. C., Shinn, M. R., Walker, H. M., et al. (2002). Selecting and evaluating classroom interventions. In *Interventions for academic and behavior problems II: Preventive and remedial approaches* (pp. 243–294). Washington, DC: National Association of School Psychologists.

Ellis, A. (1994). *Reason and emotion in psychotherapy.* New York: Harper & Row.

Ellis, A., & Bernard, M. E. (Eds.). (2006). *Rational emotive behavioral approaches to childhood disorders: Theory, practice and research.* New York: Springer.

Endress, S. A., Weston, H., Marchand-Martella, N. E., Simmons, J., & Martella, R. C. (2007). Examining the effects of Phono-Graphix on the remediation of reading skills of students with disabilities: A program evaluation. *Education and Treatment of Children, 30*(2), 1–20.

Epstein, J. L. (1995). School/family/community partnerships: Caring for the children we share. *Phi Delta Kappan, 76,* 701–412.

Esquivel, G. B., & Flanagan, R. (2007). Narrative methods of personality assessment in school psychology. *Psychology in the Schools,44,* 271–280.

Esquivel, G. B., Warren, T. M., & Olitzky, S. L (2007). In G. B. Esquivel, E. C. Lopez, & S. Nahari (Eds.), *Handbook of multicultural school psychology* (pp. 29–46). Mahwah, NJ: Erlbaum.

Exner, J. E. (2003) *The Rorschach: A comprehensive system: Vol. 1. Basic foundations* (4th ed.). Hoboken, NJ: Wiley.

Fagan, T. K. (1993). Separate but equal: School psychology's search for organizational identity. *Journal of School Psychology, 31,* 3–90.

Fagan, T. K. (2000). Practicing school psychology: A turn of the century perspective. *American Psychologist, 55,* 754–757.

Fagan, T. K. (2001). What was the most important event in school psychology's first century? *School Psychologist, 55,* 16–17.

Fagan, T. K. (2004). School psychology's significant discrepancy: Historical perspectives on personnel shortages. *Psychology in the Schools, 41*(4), 419–430.

Fagan, T. K. (2005). The 50th anniversary of the Thayer Conference: Historical perspectives and accomplishments. *School Psychology Quarterly, 20,* 224–251.

Fagan, T. K. (2008). Trends in the history of school psychology in the United States. In A. Thomas & J. Grimes (Eds.), *Best practices in school psychology* (5th ed., pp. 2069–2085). Bethesda, MD: National Association of School Psychologists.

Fagan, T. K., & Wise, P. S. (2000). *School psychology: Past, present, and future* (2nd ed.). Washington, DC: National Association of School Psychologists.

Fagan, T. K., & Wise, P. S. (2007). *School psychology: Past, present, and future* (3rd ed.). Bethesda, MD: National Association of School Psychologists.

Family Educational Rights and Privacy Act of 1974 (FERPA), part of Pub. L. No. 93–390, 20 U.S.C. § 1232g. Regulations appear at 34 C.F.R. § Part 99.

Fischetti, B. A., & Crespi, T. (1999). Clinical supervision for school psychologists. *School Psychology International, 20,* 278–288.

Fishel, M., & Ramirez, L. (2005). Evidence-based parent involvement interventions with school-aged children. *School Psychology Quarterly, 20*(4), 371–402.

Flanagan, R. (1995). A review of the Behavior Assessment System for Children: Assessment consistent with the requirements of the Individuals with Disabilities Education Act. *Journal of School Psychology, 33,* 177–186.

Flanagan, R. (2004). The Diplomate in School Psychology: Implications for the science and practice of school psychology. *Psychology in the Schools, 41,* 481–488.

Flanagan, R. (2007). Comments on the miniseries: Personality assessment in school psychology. *Psychology in the Schools, 44,* 311–318.

Flanagan, R., Allen, K., & Henry, D. (2010). A comparison of problem solving to problem solving plus rational emotive behavior therapy: An intervention to improve children's anger management. *Journal of Rational Emotive and Cognitive Behavior Therapy. 28*(2), 87–99. *DOI 10.1007/s10942-009-0102-4*

Flanagan, R., Costantino, G., Cardalda, E., & Costantino, E. (2007). TEMAS, a multicultural test and its place in an assessment battery. In L. Suzuki & J. Ponterotto (Eds.), *Handbook of multicultural assessment* (3rd ed., pp. 323–345). San Francisco: Jossey-Bass.

Flanagan, R., & Esquivel, G. (2006). Empirical and clinical methods in the assessment of personality and psychopathology: An integrative approach for training. *Psychology in the Schools, 43,* 513-526.

Flanagan, R., Miller, J. A., & Jacob, S. (2005). The 2002 revision of Ethical Principles for Psychologists: Implications for school psychologists. *Psychology in the Schools, 42,* 433–445.

Flanagan, R., & Motta, R. (2007). Figure drawings: A popular method. *Psychology in the Schools, 44,* 257–270.

Frank, L. K. (1939). Projective methods for the study of personality. *Journal of Psychology Interdisciplinary and Applied, 8,* 389–413.

Fuchs, L. S. (2003). Assessing intervention responsiveness: Conceptual and technical issues. *Learning Disabilities Research and Practice, 18,* 172–186.

Fuchs, L. S., & Deno, S. L. (1991). Paradigmatic distinctions between instructionally relevant measurement models. *Exceptional Children, 57,* 488–500.

Fuertes, J., Alfonso, V. C., & Schultz, J. T. (2007). Counseling culturally and linguistically diverse youth: A self-regulatory approach. In G. B. Esquivel, E. C. Lopez., & S. Nahari (Eds.), *Handbook of multicultural school psychology* (pp. 409–472). Mahwah, NJ: Erlbaum.

Gallo-Lopez, L. (2000). A creative play therapy approach to the group treatment of sexually abused children. In H. G. Kaduson & C. E. Schaeffer (Eds.), *Short-term play therapy for children* (pp. 269–295). New York: Guilford Press.

Garcia, M. (2004). Reflectivity in consultation. In N. M. Lambert, I. Hylander, & J. H. Sandoval (Eds.), *Consultee-centered consultation* (pp. 359-369). Mahwah, NJ: Erlbaum.

Genesee, F., Lindholm-Leary, K., Saunders, W., & Christian, D. (2005). English language learners in U.S. schools: An overview of research findings. *Journal of Education for Students Placed at Risk, 10,* 363–385.

Gettinger, M., & Stoiber, K. (2009). Effective teaching and effective schools. In T. B. Gutkin & C. R. Reynolds (Eds.), *The handbook of school psychology* (4th ed., pp. 769–790). New York: John Wiley.

Gilbertson, D., Duhon, G., Witt J. C., & Dufrene, B. (2008). Effects of academic response rates on time-on-task in the classroom for students at academic and behavioral risk. *Education & Treatment of Children, 31*(2), 153–165.

Gilliam, J. E. (2006). *Gilliam Autism Rating Scale* (2nd ed.). Austin, TX: Pro-Ed.

Goldstein, A. P. (1988). *The Prepare Curriculum: Teaching prosocial competencies.* Champaign, IL: Research Press.

Gould, S. J. (1981). *The mismeasure of man.* New York: W. W. Norton.

Graves, S. L., Jr., & Wright, L. B. (2007). Comparison of individual factors in school psychology graduate students: Why do students pursue a degree in school psychology? *Psychology in the Schools, 44*(8), 865–872.

Greenberg, M. T., Kusché, C. , & Mihalic, S. F. (1998). *Promoting Alternative Thinking Strategies (PATHS): Blueprints for violence prevention, Book Ten*. Blueprints for Violence Prevention Series (D. S. Elliott, Series Editor). Boulder, CO: Center for the Study and Prevention of Violence, Institute of Behavioral Science, University of Colorado.

Greene, J. P. (1998). A meta-analysis of the effectiveness of bilingual education. Unpublished manuscript available at www.hks.harvard.edu/pepg/PDF/Papers/biling.pdf.

Gresham, F. M. (2002). Responsiveness to intervention: An alternative approach to the identification of learning disabilities. In R. Bradley, L. Danielson, & D. Hallahan (Eds.), *Identification of learning disabilities: Research to practice* (pp. 467–519). Mahwah, NJ: Erlbaum.

Gresham, F. M., Gansle, K. A., Noell, G. H., Cohen, S., & Rosenblum, S. (1993). Treatment integrity of school-based behavioral intervention studies. *School Psychology Review, 22,* 254–272.

Gresham, F., Watson, T., & Skinner, C. H (2001). Functional behavioral assessment: Principles, procedures, and future directions. *School Psychology Review, 30*, 156–172.

Gresham, F. M., & Witt J. C. (1997). Utility of intelligence tests for treatment planning, classification and placement decisions: Recent empirical finding and future directions. *School Psychology Quarterly, 12,* 249–267.

Gutkin, T. K. (1993). Moving from behavioral to eco-behavioral consultation. What's in a name? *Journal of Educational and Psychological Consultation, 4,* 95–99.

Gutkin, T. K., & Curtis, M. J. (1999). School-based consultation theory and practice: The art and science of indirect service delivery. In C. R. Reynolds & T. K. Gutkin (Eds.), *Handbook of school psychology* (2nd ed., pp. 598–637). New York: Wiley.

Gutkin, T. B., & Reynolds, C. R. (Eds.). (2009). *The handbook of school psychology* (4th ed.). New York: John Wiley & Sons.

Guva, G.(2004). Meeting with a teacher who asks for help, but not for consultation. In N. M. Lambert, I. Hylander, & J. H. Sandoval (Eds.), *Consultee-centered consultation*. (pp. 257–266). Mahwah, NJ: Erlbaum.

Haboush, K. L. (2003). Group supervision of school psychologists in training. *School Psychology International, 24*, 232–255.

Haldeman, D. (2000). Gender identity disorder: Issues for school psychologists. *School Psychology Review, 29,* 192–200.

Hale, J. B., & Fiorello, C. A. (2004). *School neuropsychology: A practitioner's handbook*. New York: Guilford Press.

Hale, J. B., Fiorello, C. A., Kavanagh, J. A., Hoeppner, J.-A. B., & Gaither, R. A. (2001). WISC-III predictors of academic achievement for children with learning disabilities: Are global and factor scores comparable? *School Psychology Quarterly, 16*(1), 31–55.

Hall, E. T. (1966). *The hidden dimension*. Garden City, NY: Doubleday.

Hall, T. M., Kaduson, H. G., & Schaeffer, C. E. (2006). Fifteen effective play therapy techniques. *Professional Psychology: Research and Practice, 33,* 515–522.

Halstead, J. M. (2005). Religion, culture, and schooling. In C. L. Frisby & C. R. Reynolds (Eds.), *Comprehensive handbook of multicultural school psychology* (pp. 394–424). New York: Wiley.

Hannay, H. J., Bieliauskas, L. A., Crosson, B. A., Hammeke, T. A., Hamsher, K. deS., & Koffler, S. P. (1998). Proceedings of the Houston Conference on Specialty Education and Training in Clinical Neuropsychology. *Archives of Clinical Neuropsychology, 13*, 157–250.

Harvey, V. S., & Struzziero, J. (2000). *Effective supervision in school psychology*. Bethesda, MD: National Association of School Psychologists.

Hawkins, P., & Shohet, R. (2006). *Supervision in the helping professions* (3rd ed.). Berkshire, UK: Open University Press.

Health Insurance Portability and Accountability Act of 1996 (HIPAA). Pub. L. No. 104–191.

Hersen, M., & Bellack, A. S. (1981). *Behavioral assessment* (2nd ed.). New York: Pergamon Press.

Hintze, J. M. (2009). Curriculum-based assessment. In T. B. Gutkin & C. R. Reynolds (Eds.), *The handbook of school psychology* (4th ed., pp. 397–409). New York: John Wiley.

Hollander, G. (2000). Questioning youths: Challenges to working with youths forming identities. *School Psychology Review, 29,*173–179.

Hollingsworth, L. S. (1933) .Psychological service for public schools. *Teachers College Record, 34,* 368–379.

Horn, J. L., & Cattell, R. B. (1966). Refinement and test of the theory of fluid and crystallized general intelligences. *Journal of Educational Psychology, 57,* 253–270.

Hosp, J. L., & Reschly, D. J. (2002). Regional differences in school psychology practice. *School Psychology Review, 31*(1), 11–29.

Hughes, J. N. (1986). Ethical issues in school consultation. *School Psychology Review, 15,* 489–499.

Hughes, T. L., Gacono, C. B., & Owen, P. (2007). The current status of Rorschach assessment in school psychology. *Psychology in the Schools, 44,* 281–292.

Hughes, T. L., Kaufman, J., & Miller, J. A. (2010). Is everything old new again: School psychology training past, present, and future. In J. Kaufman, T. L. Hughes, & C. Riccio (Eds.), *Handbook of education, training and supervision of school psychologists in school and community (pp. 3-15).* New York: Routledge.

Hughes, T. L., & Morine, K. (2005, August). *Using creative and critical thinking for psychological report writing.* Paper presented at the American Psychological Association annual conference, Washington, DC.

Hughes, T. L., & Theodore, L. A. (2009). Conceptual frame for selecting individual psychotherapy in the schools. *Psychology in the Schools, 46,* 218–224.

Hunsley, J. (2007). Addressing key challenges in evidence-based practice in psychology. *Professional Psychology: Research and Practice, 38*(2), 113–121.

Hylander, I. (2004a). Analysis of conceptual change in consultee-centered consultation. In N. M. Lambert, I. Hylander, & J. H. Sandoval (Eds.), *Consultee-centered consultation* (pp. 45–61). Mahwah, NJ: Erlbaum.

Hylander, I. (2004b). Identifying change in consultee-centered consultation. In N. M. Lambert, I. Hylander, & J. H. Sandoval (Eds.), *Consultee-centered consultation* (pp. 373–389). Mahwah, NJ: Erlbaum.

Individuals with Disabilities Education Act (IDEA). Pub. L. No. 101– 476, 20 U.S.C. Chapter 33.Amended by Pub. L. No. 106–17 in June 1997. Regulations appear at 34 C.F.R. Part 300.

Individuals with Disabilities Education Improvement Act (IDEIA). Pub.L. No. 108–446, 20, U.S.C., 1400-87 (2004). Regulations appear at 34 C.F.R. Part 300.

Ingraham, C. (2004). Multicultural consultee-centered consultation: supporting consultees in the development of cultural competence. In N. M. Lambert, I. Hylander, & J. H. Sandoval (Eds.), *Consultee-centered consultation* (pp. 133-148). Mahwah, NJ: Erlbaum.

Inhelder, B. , & Piaget, J. (1958). *The Growth of Logical Thinking from Childhood to Adolescence.* New York: Basic Books.

Ivey, A. E., & Ivey, M. B. (2007). *Intentional interviewing and counseling* (6th ed.). Belmont, CA: Thomson.

Ivey, A. E., & Ivey, M. B. (2008). *Essentials of intentional interviewing*. Belmont, CA: Brooks-Cole.

Izard, C. E., King, K. A., Trentacosta, C. J., Laurenceau, J.-P., Finlon, K. J., Krauthamer-Ewing, E. S., et al. (2008). Accelerating the development of emotion competence in Head Start children: Effects on adaptive and maladaptive behavior. *Development and Psychopathology, 20*(1), 369–397.

Jacob K. Javits Gifted and Talented Students Education Act of 1988. Pub. L. No. 100-297. Available at www.ed.gov/policy/elsec/leg/esea02/pg72.html.

Jacob, S., & Hartshorne, T. (2007). *Ethics and law for school psychologists* (5th ed.). Hoboken, NJ: Wiley.

Johannessen, E. M. (2004). Complicating the thinking of the consultee. In N. M. Lambert, I. Hylander, & J. H. Sandoval (Eds.), *Consultee-centered consultation* (pp. 247–253). Mahwah, NJ: Erlbaum.

Kaduson, H. G., & Schaeffer, C. E. (2000). *Short-term play therapy for children*. New York: Guilford Press.

Kam, C.-M., Greenberg, M. T., & Kusché, C. A. (2004). Sustained effects of the PATHS curriculum on the social and psychological adjustment of children in special education. *Journal of Emotional and Behavioral Disorders, 12*(2), 66–78.

Kaminski, R. A., Cummings, K. D., Powell-Smith, K. A., & Good, R. H. I. (2008). Best practices in using Dynamic Indicators of Basic Early Literacy skills for formative assessment and evaluation. In A. Thomas & J. Grimes (Eds.), *Best practices in school psychology V* (Vol. 4, pp. 1181–1203). Bethesda, MD: National Association of School Psychologists.

Kaminski, R. A., & Good, R. H. III. (1996). Toward a technology for assessing basic early literacy skills. *School Psychology Review, 25*(2), 215–227.

Kamphaus, R. (1998). *School psychology: Prospective and retrospective views of the field* (pp. 13–18). Alfred, NY: Lea R. Powell Institute for Children and Families.

Kamphaus, R. W. (2009). Assessment of intelligence and achievement. In T. B. Gutkin & C. R. Reynolds (Eds.), *The handbook of school psychology* (4th ed., pp. 230–246). New York: John Wiley.

Kane, H. & Boan, C. H. (2005). A review and critique of multicultural learning styles. In C. L. Frisby & C. R. Reynolds (Eds.), *Comprehensive handbook of multicultural school psychology* (pp. 425–456). New York: Wiley.

Kaslow, N. J. (2004). Competencies in professional psychology. *American Psychologist, 59,* 774–781.

Kaslow, N. J., Rubin, N. J., Bebeau, M. J., Leigh, I. W., Lichtenberg, J. W., Nelson, P. D., Portnoy, S. M., & Smith, I. L. (2007). Guiding principles for the assessment and recommendation of competence. *Professional Psychology: Research and Practice, 38,* 441–451.

Kaufman, A. S., & Kaufman, N. L. (2004a). *Kaufman Assessment Battery for Children* (2nd ed.). Circle Pines, MN: AGS Publishing.

Kaufman, A. S., & Kaufman, N. L. (2004b). *Kaufman Test of Educational* Achievement (2nd ed.). Circle Pines, MN: American Guidance Service.

Kazdin, A. E. (1980). Acceptability of alternative treatments for deviant child behavior. *Journal of Applied Behavior Analysis, 13*(2), 259–273.

Kazdin, A. E. (2001). *Behavior modification* (6th ed.). Belmont, CA: Wadsworth.

Kazdin, A. E., & Weisz, J.R., (2003). *Evidence-based psychotherapies for children and adolescents.* New York: Guilford Press.

Keith, T. Z. (1998). School psychology: A good and plausible future. In E. Gaughan & E. Faherty (Eds.), *School psychology: Prospective and retrospective views of the field* (pp. 13–18). Alfred, NY: Lea R. Powell Institute for Children and Families.

Keith, T. Z., & Fine, J. G. (2005). Multicultural influences on school learning: Similarities and differences across groups. In C. L. Frisby & C. R. Reynolds (Eds.), *Comprehensive handbook of multicultural school psychology* (pp. 425–456.). New York: Wiley.

Kelley-Laine, K. (1998). Parents as partners in schooling: The current state of affairs. *Childhood Education, 74*(6), 342–345.

Kendall, P. C., Aschenbrand, S. G., & Hudson, J. H. (2003). Child-focused treatment of anxiety. In A. E. Kazdin & J. R. Weisz (Eds.), *Evidence-based psychotherapies for children and adolescents* (pp. 81–100). New York: Guilford Press.

Knapp, M. L., & Hall, J. (1997). *Nonverbal communication in human interaction* (5th ed.). Orlando, FL: Holt, Reinhart, & Winston.

Knapp, S., & VandeCreek, L. (2003). An overview of the major changes in the 2002 APA ethics code. *Professional Psychology: Research and Practice, 34,* 301–308.

Knapp, S. J., & VandeCreek, L. D. (2006). *Practical ethics for psychologists.* Washington, DC: American Psychological Association.

Knell, S. M. (1998). Cognitive-behavioral play therapy. *Journal of Child Clinical Psychology, 27,* 28–33.

Knotek, S. (2004). Developing through discourse: Speech genres as pathways to conceptualization change. In N. M. Lambert, I. Hylander, & J. H. Sandoval (Eds.), *Consultee-centered consultation* (pp. 351–360). Mahwah, NJ: Erlbaum.

Kogan, E. (2001). *Gifted bilingual students: A paradox?* New York: Peter Lang.

Korkman, M., Kirk, U., & Kemp, S. (2007). *NEPSY-II.* San Antonio, TX: Psychological Corporation.

Kovacs, M. (1992). *Children's Depression Inventory.* North Tonawanda, NY: Multi-Health Systems.

Kratochwill, T. R. (1977). N=1: An alternative research strategy for school psychologists. *Psychology in the Schools, 15,* 239–249.

Kratochwill, T. R. (2005). Theories of change and adoption of innovations: The evolving evidence-based intervention and practice movement in school psychology. *Psychology in the Schools, 42,* 475–494.

Kratochwill, T. R., Eaton Hoagwood, K., Mass Levitt, J., Olin, S., Frank, J. L., & Saka, N. (2009). Evidence-based interventions and practices in school psychology: Challenges and opportunities for the profession. In T. B. Gutkin & C. R. Reynolds (Eds.), *The handbook of school psychology* (4th ed., pp. 497–521). New York: John Wiley.

Kratochwill, T. R., Elliott, S. N., & Stoiber, K. C. (2002). Best practices in school-based problem-solving consultation. In A. Thomas & J. Grimes (Eds.), *Best practices in school psychology IV* (pp. 583–608). Bethesda, MD: National Association of School Psychologists.

Kratochwill, T. R., & Stoiber, K. C. (2000a). Empirically supported interventions and school psychology: Conceptual and practice issues—Part II. *School Psychology Quarterly, 15*(2), 233–253.

Kratochwill, T. R., & Stoiber, K. C. (2000b). Diversifying theory and science: Expanding the boundaries of empirically supported interventions in school psychology. *Journal of School Psychology, 38*(4), 349–358.

Kuhn, T. (1962). *The structure of scientific revolutions.* Chicago: Chicago University Press.

Lachar, D., & Gruber, C. P. (1994). *Personality Inventory for Youth.* Los Angeles, CA: Western Psychological Services.

Lachar, D., & Wirt, R. D. (2001). *Personality Inventory for Children.* Los Angeles, CA: Western Psychological Services.

Lambert, N. M. (1981). Psychological evidence in Larry P. vs. Wilson Riles: An evaluation by a witness for the defense. *American Psychologist, 36,* 937–952.

Lambert, N. M. (1986). Conceptual foundations for school psychology: Perspectives from the development of the school psychology program at Berkeley. *Professional School Psychology, 1,* 215–223.

Lambert, N. M. (2004). Consultee-centered consultation: An international perspective on goals, process and theory. In N. M. Lambert, I. Hylander, & J. H. Sandoval (Eds.), *Consultee-centered consultation* (pp. 3– 20). Mahwah, NJ: Erlbaum.

Lambert, N. M., Hylander, I., & Sandoval, J. H. (Eds.). (2004). *Consultee-centered consultation.* Mahwah, NJ: Erlbaum.

Leech, N. L., & Onwuegbuzie, A. J. (2008). Qualitative data analysis: A compendium of techniques and a framework for selection for school psychology research and beyond. *School Psychology Quarterly, 23,* 587–604.

Lochman, J. E., Barry, T. D., & Pardini, D. A. (2003). Anger control training for aggressive youth. In A. E. Kazdin, & J. R. Weisz (Eds.), *Evidence-based psychotherapies for children and adolescents* (pp. 241–262). New York: Guilford Press.

Lopez, E. C. (2002). Best practices in working with school interpreters to deliver psychological services to children and families. In A. Thomas & J. Grimes (Eds.), *Best practices in school psychology* (4th ed., pp. 1419–1432). Bethesda, MD: National Association of School Psychologists.

Matarazzo, J. D. (1987). There is only one psychology, no specialties, but many applications. *American Psychologist, 42*(10), 893–903.

Mather, N., & Jaffe, L. E. (2002). *Woodcock-Johnson III: Reports, recommendations, and strategies.* New York: John Wiley.

McCabe, P. C., & Rubinson, F. (2008). Committing to social justice: The behavioral intention of school psychology and education trainees to advocate for lesbian, gay, bisexual and transgendered youth. *School Psychology Review, 37,*469–486.

McCallum, E., Skinner, C. H., Turner, H., & Saecker, L. (2006). The taped-problems intervention: Increasing multiplication fact fluency using a low-tech, classwide, time-delay intervention. *School Psychology Review, 35*(3), 419–434.

McGuinness, C., McGuinness, D., & McGuinness, G. (1996). Phono-Graphix: A new method for remediating reading difficulties. *Annals of Dyslexia, 46,* 73–96.

McGrew, K. S., & Flanagan, D. (1998). *The intelligence test desk reference: Gf-Gc cross-battery assessment.* Needham Heights, MA: Allyn & Bacon.

McGrew, M. W., & Teglasi, H. (1990). Formal characteristics of the Thematic Apperception Test stories as indices of emotional disturbance in children. *Journal of Personality Assessment, 54,* 639–655.

McIntosh, D. E. (2004). Addressing the shortage of school psychologists: Introduction. *Psychology in the Schools, 41*(4), 411–413.

McIntosh, D. E., & Phelps, L. (2000). Supervision in school psychology: Where will the future take us? *Psychology in the Schools, 37,* 33–38.

210 *References*

McIntosh, D. N., & Spilka, B. (1998). Religion and the family. In B. R. Neff & D. Ratcliff (Eds.), *Handbook of family religious education* (pp. 36–60). Birmingham, AL: Religious Education Press.

Mead, D. E. (1990). *Effective supervision.* New York: Brunner Mazel.

Medway, F. (1979). How effective is school consultation? A review of recent research. *Journal of School Psychology, 17,* 272–282.

Mercer, S. H., & DeRosier, M. E. (2008). Teacher preference, peer rejection, and student aggression: A prospective study of transactional influence and independent contributions to emotional adjustment and grades. *Journal of School Psychology, 46*(6), 661–685.

Merrell, K. W., Ervin, R., & Gimpel, G. A. (2006). *School psychology for the 21st century: Foundations and practices.* New York: Guilford Press.

Messick, S. (1995). Validity of psychological assessment: Validation of inferences from persons' responses and performances as scientific inquiry into score meaning. *American Psychologist, 50,* 741–749.

Meyers, J., & Nastasi, B. K. (1999). Primary prevention in school settings. In C. R. Reynolds & T. B. Gutkin (Eds.), *The handbook of school psychology* (3rd ed., pp. 764–799). New York: John Wiley.

Miller, D. C. (2007). *Essentials of school neuropsychological assessment.* Hoboken, NJ: John Wiley.

Miller, D. C. (Ed.). (2010), *Best practices in school neuropsychology.* Hoboken, NJ: John Wiley.

Miller, J. A., & Leffard, S. A. (2007). Behavioral assessment. In S. R. Smith & L. Handler (Eds.), *The clinical assessment of children and adolescents: A practitioner's handbook* (pp. 115–137). Mahwah, NJ: Erlbaum.

Miller, J.,A., Tansy, M., & Hughes, T. L. (1998). Functional behavioral assessment: The link between problem behavior and effective intervention in the schools. *Current Issues in Education, 1.* Available at http://cie.ed.asu.edu.

Miller, L. K. (1975). *Principles of everyday behavior analysis.* Monterey, CA: Brooks-Cole.

Minke, K. M., & Brown, D. T. (1996). Preparing psychologists to work with children: A comparison of curricula in child-clinical and school psychology programs. *Professional Psychology: Research and Practice, 27*(6), 631–634.

Miranda, A. H., & Gutter, P. B. (2002). Diversity research literature in school psychology, 1990–1999. *Psychology in the Schools, 39,* 597–604.

Murray, H. M. (1943). *Thematic Apperception Test.* Cambridge, MA: Harvard University Press.

Nagle, R. J., Suldo, S. M., Christenson, S. L., & Hansen, A. L. (2004). Graduate students' perspectives of academic positions in school psychology. *School Psychology Quarterly, 19*(4), 311–326.

Naglieri, J. A., & Das, J. P. (1997). *Cognitive Assessment System.* Itasca, IL: Riverside.

National Association of School Psychologists (NASP). (1997). *The principles for professional ethics.* Bethesda, MD: Author.

National Association of School Psychologists (NASP). (2000a). *Principles for professional ethics, Guidelines for provision of school psychological services.* Professional Conduct Manual (pp. 13–62). Retrieved February 4, 2009, from www.nasponline.org.

National Association of School Psychologists (NASP). (2000b). *Standards for training and field placement programs in school psychology. Standards for the credentialing of school psychologists.* Retrieved February 4, 2009, from www.nasponline.org.

National Association of School Psychologists (NASP). (2003). *Who are school psychologists?* Retrieved May 10, 2008, from www.nasponline.org.

National Association of School Psychologists (NASP). (2006). *School psychology: A blueprint for training and practice* (3rd. ed.). Retrieved May 10, 2008 from National Association of School Psychologists Web site: www.nasponline.org/resources/blueprint/.

National Clearinghouse for English Language Acquisition. (2008). *The growing numbers of limited English proficient students 1996/96-2005/06.* Retrieved October 18, 2008, from www.ncela.gwu.edu.

National Institute of Child Health and Human Development. (2000). *Health disparities: Bridging the gap.* Rockville, MD: Author.

New Freedom Commission on Mental Health. (2003). *Achieving the promise: Transforming mental health care in America. Final Report* (DHHS Publication No. SMA-03-3832). Rockville, MD: Substance Abuse and Mental Health Services Administration, Center for Mental Health Service.

Nezu, A. M., Nezu, C. M., & Cos, T. A. (2007). Case formulation for the behavioral and cognitive therapies. In T. D. Eells (Ed.) , *Handbook of psychotherapy case formulation* (2nd ed., pp. 349–378). New York: Guilford Press.

No Child Left Behind Act of 2001 (NCLB). Pub.L. No. 107-110. Available at www.ed.gov.

Noell, G., & Gansle, K. (2006). Assuring the form has substance: Treatment plan implementation as the foundation of assessing Response to Intervention. *Assessment for Effective Intervention, 32,* 32–39.

Noell, G. H., Witt J. C., Slider, N. J., Connell, J. E., Gatti, S. L., Williams, K. L., Koenig, J. L., Resetar, J. L., & Duhon, G. J. (2005). Treatment implementation following behavioral consultation: A comparison of three follow-up strategies. *School Psychology Review,34,* 87–106.

Oades-Sese, V., Esquivel, G. B., & Anon, C. (2007). Identifying gifted and talented culturally and linguistically diverse children and adolescents. In G. B. Esquivel, E. C. Lopez., & S. Nahari (Eds.), *Handbook of multicultural school psychology* (pp. 453–477). Mahwah, NJ: Erlbaum.

Overstreet, S., & Braun, S. (1999). A preliminary examination of the relationship between exposure to community violence and academic functioning. *School Psychology Quarterly, 14,* 380–396.

Perusse, R., Goodnough, G. E., & Lee, V.V. (2009). Group counseling in the schools. *Psychology in the Schools, 46,* 225–231.

Phelps. L. (1998). *Health-related disorders in children and adolescents.* Washington, DC: American Psychological Association.

Phelps, L. (2005). Health-related issues among ethnic minority and low-income children: Psychoeducational outcomes and prevention models. In C. R. Frisby & C. R. Reynolds (Eds.), *Comprehensive handbook of multicultural school psychology* (pp. 928– 944). Hoboken, NJ: Wiley.

Phelps, L., McGrew, K. S., Knopik, S. N., & Ford, L. (2005). The general (g), broad, and narrow CHC stratum characteristics of the WJ III and WISC-III tests: A confirmatory cross-battery investigation. *School Psychology Quarterly, 20,* 66–88.

Piers, E. V., Harris, D. B., & Herzberg, D. S. (2002). *Manual for the Piers-Harris Self-Concept Scale for Children.* Los Angeles: Western Psychological Services.

Power, T. J. (2002). Preparing school psychologists as interventionists and preventionists. In M. R. Shinn, H. M. Walker, & G. Stoner (Eds.), *Interventions for academic and behavioral problems II: Preventive and remedial approaches* (pp. 1047–1065). Bethesda, MD: National Association of School Psychologists.

Power, T. J., DuPaul, G., Shapiro, E. S., & Parrish, J. M. (1998). Role of the school-based professional in health-related services. In L. Phelps (Ed.), *Health-related disorders in children and adolescents* (pp. 15–26). Washington, DC: American Psychological Association.

Pressley, M., Duke, N. K., Fingeret, L., Park, Y., Reffitt, K., Mohan, L., et al. (2009). Working with struggling readers: Why we must get beyond the simple view of reading and visions of how it might be done. In T. B. Gutkin & C. R. Reynolds (Eds.), *The handbook of school psychology* (4th ed., pp. 522–546). New York: John Wiley.

Prochaska, J. O., & DiClemente, C. C. (2003). The transtheoretical approach. In J. C. Norcross & M. R. Goldfried (Eds.), *Handbook of psychotherapy integration* (2nd ed., pp. 147–171). New York: Oxford University Press.

Proctor, B. E., & Steadman, T. (2003). Job satisfaction, burnout, and perceived effectiveness of "in-house" versus traditional school psychologists. *Psychology in the Schools, 40*(2), 237–243.

Ramo, J. C. (2009). *The age of the unthinkable: Why the new world disorder constantly surprises us and what we can do about it.* New York: Little, Brown.

Raskin, N. N. J., & Rogers, C. R. (1989). Person-centered therapy. In R. J. Corsini, & D. Wedding (Eds.), *Current psychotherapies* (4th ed., pp. 155–194). Itasca, IL: Peacock Press.

Reis, S. M., & Renzulli, J. S. (2004). Current research and the social and emotional development of gifted and talented students: Good news and future possibilities. *Psychology in the Schools, 41,* 119–130.

Rehabilitation Act of 1973. Pub.L. No. 93-112, 29 U.S.C. 794. Regulations implementing Section 504 appear at 34 C.F.R. Part 104 (1996).

Renzulli, J. S. (1978). What makes giftedness: Reexamining a definition. *Phi Delta Kappan, 60,* 180–184.

Reschly, D. J. (1997). Utility of individual ability measures and public policy choices for the 21st century. *School Psychology Review, 26*(2), 234–241.

Reschly, D. J. (2000). The present and future status of school psychology in the United States. *School Psychology Review, 29,* 507–522.

Reschly, D. J. (2008). School psychology paradigm shift and beyond. In A. Thomas & J. Grimes (Eds.), *Best practices in school psychology* (5th ed., pp. 3–16). Bethesda, MD: National Association of School Psychologists.

Reschly, D. J., & Wilson, M. S. (1995). School psychology practitioners and faculty: 1986 to 1991–1992: Trends in demographics, roles, satisfaction, and system reform. *School Psychology Review, 24,* 62–80.

Reynolds, C. R., & Carson, A. D. (2005). Methods for assessing cultural bias in tests. In C. R. Frisby & C. R. Reynolds (Eds.), *Comprehensive handbook of multicultural school psychology* (pp. 795–823). Hoboken, NJ: Wiley.

Reynolds, C. R., & Fletcher-Janzen , E. (2007). *Encyclopedia of special education* (3rd ed.). Hoboken, NJ: Wiley.

Reynolds, C. R., Gutkin, T. B., Elliott, S. N., & Witt J. C. (1984). *School psychology: Essentials of theory and practice.* New York: John Wiley.

Reynolds, C. R., & Kamphaus, R. W. (2003). *Reynolds Intellectual Assessment Scales.* Lutz, FL: Psychological Assessment Resources.

Reynolds, C. R., & Kamphaus, R. W. (2004). *Behavior Assessment System for Children* (2nd ed.). Minneapolis, MN: Pearson.

Reynolds, C. R., & Lowe, P. A. (2009). The problem of bias in psychological assessment. In T. B. Gutkin & C. R. Reynolds (Eds.), *The handbook of school psychology* (4th ed., pp. 332–374). New York: John Wiley.

Reynolds, C. R., & Richmond, B. O. (2008). *Revised Children's Manifest Anxiety Scale* (2nd ed.). Los Angeles: Western Psychological Services.

Reynolds, C. R., & Shaywitz S. E. (2009). Response to intervention: Ready or not? Or, from wait-to-fail to watch-them-fail. *School Psychology Quarterly, 24,* 130–145.

Reynolds, C., & Voress, J. K. (2007). *Test of Memory and Learning* (2nd ed.). Austin, TX: PRO-ED.

Riccio, C. A., & Rodriguez, O. L. (2007). Integration of psychological assessment approaches in school psychology. *Psychology in the Schools, 44,* 243–255.

Rice, V. J., & Duncan, J. R. (2006). What does it mean to be a "professional" . . . and what does it mean to be an ergonomics professional? Retrieved July, 2007, from www.ergofoundation.org/FPE1_Professionalism.pdf.

Riggs, N. R., Greenberg, M. T., Kusché, C. A., & Pentz, M. A. (2006). The mediational role of neurocognition in the behavioral outcomes of a social-emotional prevention program in elementary school students: Effects of the PATHS curriculum. *Prevention Science, 7*(1), 91–102.

Rittel, H., & Webber, M. (1973). Dilemmas in a general theory of planning. *Policy Sciences, 4*(2), 155–169.

Robin, A. L. (2003). Behavioral family systems therapy for adolescents with anorexia nervosa. In A. E. Kazdin, & J. R. Weisz (Eds.), *Evidence-based psychotherapies for children and adolescents* (pp. 358–373). New York: Guilford Press.

Robbins, M. S., Szapocznik, J., Santisteban, D. A., Hervis, O. E., Mitrani, V. B., & Schwartz, S. J. (2003). Brief strategic family therapy for Hispanic youth. In A. E. Kazdin & J. R.Weisz (Eds.), *Evidence-based psychotherapies for children and adolescents* (pp. 407–424). New York: Guilford Press.

Roberts, G. E., & Gruber, C. (2007). *Roberts-2.* Los Angeles, CA: Western Psychological Services.

Rodolfa, E., Bent, R., Eisman, E., Nelson, P., Rehm, L., & Ritchie, P. (2005). A cube model for competency development: Implications for psychology educators and regulators. *Professional Psychology: Research and Practice, 36,* 347–354.

Rogers, C. , Gendlin, E., Kiesler, D. , & Truax, C. (1967). *The therapeutic relationship ands its impact: A study of psychotherapy with schizophrenics.* Madison, WI: University of Wisconsin Press.

Roid, G. H. (2003). *Stanford-Binet Intelligence Scales* (5th ed.), *Technical Manual.* Itasca, IL: Riverside.

Rosenfield, S. (1987). *Instructional consultation.* Mahwah, NJ: Erlbaum.

Rosenfield, S. (2002a). Best practices in instructional consultation. In A. Thomas & J. Grimes (Eds.), *Best practices in school psychology* (4th ed., pp. 609–624). Bethesda, MD: National Association of School Psychologists.

Rosenfield, S. (2002b) Developing instructional consultants: From novice to competent to expert. *Journal of Educational and Psychological Consultation, 13,* 97–111.

Rosenfield, S. (2004). Consultation as dialogue: The right words at the right time. In N. M. Lambert, I. Hylander, & J. H. Sandoval (Eds.), *Consultee-centered consultation* (pp. 337–347). Mahwah, NJ: Erlbaum.

Ryan, D., & Martin, A. (2000). Lesbian, gay, bisexual, and transgender parents in the school systems. *School Psychology Review, 29,* 207–216.

Ryan-Arredondo, K., & Sandoval, J. (2005). Psychometric issues in the measurement of acculturation. In C. R. Frisby & C. R. Reynolds (Eds.), *Comprehensive handbook of multicultural school psychology* (pp. 861–880). Hoboken, NJ: Wiley.

Sadoski, M., & Willson, V. L. (2006). Effects of a theoretically based large-scale reading intervention in a multicultural urban school district. *American Educational Research Journal, 43*(1), 137–154.

Sandoval, J. H. (2004a). Conceptual change in consultee-centered consultation. In N. M. Lambert, I. Hylander, & J. H. Sandoval (Eds.), *Consultee-centered consultation* (pp. 37–44). Mahwah, NJ: Erlbaum.

Sandoval, J. H. (2004b). Evaluation issues and strategies in consultee-centered consultation. In N. M. Lambert, I. Hylander, & J. H. Sandoval (Eds.), *Consultee-centered consultation* (pp. 393–400). Mahwah, NJ: Erlbaum.

Sattler, J. M. (1998). Clinical and forensic interviewing of children and families. San Diego: Author.

Sattler, J.M. (2001). *Assessment of children: Cognitive applications.* (4th ed.) San Diego, CA: Author.

Sattler, J. M. (2002). Assessment of children: Behavioral and clinical applications (4th ed.). San Diego, CA: Author.

Sattler, J. M. (2008). *Assessment of children: Cognitive approaches* (5th ed.). San Diego: Author.

Schaeffer, C. E. (Ed.). (1993). *The therapeutic powers of play.* Northvale, NJ: Jason Aronson.

Schopler, E., Reichler, R. J., & Renner, R. R. (1988). *Child Autism Rating Scale.* Los Angeles: Western Psychological Services.

Schrank, F. A., Miller, J., Caterino, L. C., & Desrochers, J. C. (2006). American Academy of School Psychology survey on the independent educational evaluation for a specific learning disability: Results and discussion. *Psychology in the Schools, 43*(7), 771–780.

Schrank, F. A., Wendling B. J., & Woodcock R. W. (2008). *Woodcock Interpretation and Instructional Interventions Program.* Rolling Meadows, IL: Riverside.

Schrank, F., Wolf, I. L., Flanagan, R., Reynolds, C. R., Caterino, L. C., Hyman, I. A., Miller, J. A., Swerdlik, M. E., & Davis, R. A. (2004). Statement on comprehensive evaluation for learning disabilities. *Communiqué, 32(7),* 12; republished in the *Trainer's Forum, 23*(4), 13–15.

Shapiro, E. S. (2008). Best practices in setting progress monitoring goals for academic skill improvement. In A. Thomas & J. Grimes (Eds.), *Best practices in school psychology* (5th ed., pp. 141–157). Bethesda, MD: National Association of School Psychologists.

Shaywitz S. E. (2003). *Overcoming dyslexia: A new and complete science-based program for reading problems at any level.* New York: Alfred A. Knopf.

Sheridan, S. S. (2000). Considerations of multiculturalism and diversity in behavioral consultation with parents and teachers. *School Psychology Review, 29,* 344–353.

Sheslow, D., & Adams, W. (2003). *Wide range assessment of memory and learning* (2nd ed.). Lutz, FL: Psychological Assessment Resources.

Shure, M. B. (1992a). *I Can Problem Solve: An interpersonal cognitive problem-solving program: Intermediate elementary grades.* Champaign, IL: Research Press.

Shure, M. B. (1992b). *I Can Problem Solve: An interpersonal cognitive problem-solving program: Kindergarten & primary grades.* Champaign, IL: Research Press.

Shure, M. B. (1992c). *I Can Problem Solve: An interpersonal cognitive problem-solving program: Preschool.* Champaign, IL: Research Press.

Shure, M. B. (2001). I can problem solve (ICPS): An interpersonal cognitive problem solving program for children. *Residential Treatment for Children & Youth, 18*(3), 3–14.

Siegler, R. S., & Kotovsky, K. (1986). *Conceptions of giftedness.* Cambridge, UK: Cambridge University Press.

Silva, F. (1993). *Psychometric foundations and behavioral assessment.* Newbury Park, CA: Sage.

Skinner, B. F. (1957). *Verbal behavior.* Englewood Cliffs, NJ: Prentice-Hall.

Smith, S. R., & Handler, L. (2007). *The clinical assessment of children and adolescents: A practitioner's handbook.* Mahwah, NJ: Lawrence Erlbaum.

Sparrow, S. S., Balla, D. A., & Cicchetti, D. V.(1984). *Vineland Adaptive Behavior Scales.* Circle Pines, MN: American Guidance Service.

Spearman, C. (1904). "General intelligence," objectively determined and measured. *American Journal of Psychology, 15,* 201–293.

Steege, M. W., & Harper, D. C. (1989). Enhancing the management of secondary encopresis by assessing acceptability of treatment: A case study. *Journal of Behavior Therapy and Experimental Psychiatry, 20,* 333–341.

Stephens, K. R., & Karnes, F. A. (2000). State definitions for the gifted and talented revisited. *Exceptional Children, 66,* 219–238.

Stokes, T. F., & Baer, D. M. (1977). An implicit technology of generalization. *Journal of Applied Behavior Analysis, 10,* 349–368.

Stoltenberg, C. D. (1981) Approaching supervision from a developmental perspective: The counselor complexity model. *Journal of Counseling Psychology, 31,* 3–12.

Stoltenberg, C. D. (1993). Supervising consultants in training, *Journal of Counseling and Development, 72, 131–138.*

Stoltenberg, C. D., & Delworth, U. (1987). *Supervising counselors and therapists: A developmental approach.* San Francisco: Jossey-Bass.

Stoolmiller, M., Eddy, J. M., & Reid, J. B. (2000). Detecting and describing preventive intervention effects in a universal school-based randomized trial targeting delinquent and violent behavior. *Journal of Consulting and Clinical Psychology, 68*(2), 296–306.

Stricker, G., & Trierweiler, S. J. (1995). The local clinical scientist: A bridge between science and practice. *American Psychologist, 50*(12), 995–1002.

Strong, S. R. (1968). Counseling: An interpersonal influence process. *Journal of Counseling Psychology, 15,* 215–224.

Talley, R. C., & Short, R. J. (1995). *School health: Psychology's role.* Washington, DC: American Psychological Association.

Teglasi, H. (1998). Assessment of schema and problem solving strategies with projective techniques. In C. R. Reynolds (Ed.), *Comprehensive clinical psychology: Vol. 4. Assessment* (pp. 459–499). New York: Elsevier.

Teglasi, H. (2001). *Essentials of TAT and Story Telling Techniques assessment.* New York: Wiley.

Teglasi, H. (2007) Personality assessment: The whole and its parts: Introduction to the series. *Psychology in the Schools, 44,* 209–214.

Teglasi, H., & Rothman, L. (2001). STORIES: A classroom based program to reduce aggressive behavior. *Journal of School Psychology, 39,* 71–94.

Teglasi, H., Simcox, A. G., & Kim, N. (2007) Personality constructs and measures. *Psychology in the Schools, 44,* 215–228.

Telzrow, C. F. (1995). Best practices in ensuring treatment adherence. In A. Thomas & J. Grimes (Eds.), *Best practices in school psychology* (3rd ed., pp. 501–518). Washington, DC: National Association of School Psychologists.

Telzrow, C. F., McNamara, K., & Hollinger, C. (2000). Fidelity of problem solving implementation and relationship to student performance. *School Psychology Review, 29,* 443–461.

Tharinger, D., & Perfect M. (2005). Psychotherapy. In S. W. Lee (Ed.), *Encyclopedia of school psychology* (pp. 416–420). Thousand Oaks, CA; Sage.

Tharinger, D. J., Pryzwansky, W. B., & Miller, J.A (2008). School psychology: A specialty of professional psychology with distinct competencies and complexities. *Professional Psychology: Research and Practice, 39,* 529–536.

Tharinger, D., & Wells, G. (2000). An attachment perspective on the developmental challenges of gay, lesbian and bisexual youth. *School Psychology Review, 29,*158–172.

Thomas, A., & Grimes, J. (Eds.). (2008). *Best practices in school psychology V* (5th ed.). Washington, DC: National Association of School Psychologists.

Thomas, W. P., & Collier, V. P. (1998). Two languages are better than one. *Educational Leadership, 55,* 23–27.

Thompson, B. (2003). Understanding reliability and coefficient alpha, really. In B. Thompson (Ed.), *Score reliability.* Thousand Oaks: Sage.

Thorn, S. (2004). Allowing ambiguity and listening to the contradictions. In N. M. Lambert, I. Hylander, & J. H. Sandoval (Eds.), *Consultee-centered consultation* (pp. 281–292). Mahwah, NJ: Erlbaum.

Tilly, W. D. (2008). The evolution of school psychology to science-based practice: Problem solving and the three-tiered model. In A. Thomas & J. Grimes (Eds.), *Best practices in school psychology V* (Vol. 1, pp. 17–36). Bethesda, MD: National Association of School Psychologists.

Tilly, W. D., & Flugum, K. R. (1995). Best practices in ensuring quality interventions. In A. Thomas & J. Grimes (Eds.), *Best practices in school psychology* (3rd ed., pp. 485–500). Washington, DC: National Association of School Psychologists.

Trachtman, G. M. (1981). On such a full sea. *School Psychology Review, 10*(2), 138–181.

Trager, G. L. (1958). Paralanguage: A first approximation. *Studies in Linguistics, 13,* 1–12.

Upah, K. (2008). Best practices in designing, implementing, and evaluating quality interventions. In A. Thomas & J. Grimes (Eds.), *Best practices in school psychology* (5th ed., pp. 209–223). Bethesda, MD: National Association of School Psychologists.

Upah, K., & Tilly, W. D. (2002). Best practices in designing, implementing and evaluating quality interventions. In A. Thomas & J. Grimes (Eds.), *Best practices in school psychology IV* (pp. 483–502). Bethesda, MD: National Association of School Psychologists.

U.S. Department of Education. (2006). Federal Register 34 CFR parts 300 & 301. Assistance to states for education of children with disabilities and preschool grants for children with disabilities: Final Rule, August 14, 2007.

U. S. Department of Health and Human Services. (1999). *Mental health: A report of the surgeon general.* Rockville, MD: Substance Abuse and Mental Health Services Administration, Center for Mental Health Service.

Vaden-Kiernan, N., and McManus, J. (2005). Parent and family involvement in education: 2002–03 (NCES 2005–043). U.S. Department of Education, National Center for Education Statistics. Washington, DC: U.S. Government Printing Office.

VanDerHeyden, A., & Burns, M. (2005). Effective instruction for at-risk minority populations. In C. R. Frisby & C. R. Reynolds (Eds.), *Comprehensive handbook of multicultural school psychology* (pp. 483–513). Hoboken, NJ: Wiley.

VanDerHeyden, A., & Witt J. C. (2008). Best practices in can't do/won't do assessment. In A. Thomas & J. Grimes (Eds.), *Best practices in school psychology* (5th ed., pp. 131–140). Bethesda, MD: National Association of School Psychologists.

Vane, J.R. (1985). School psychology: To be or not to be. *Journal of School Psychology, 23,* 101–112.

VanVoorhis, R. W., & Levinson, E. M. (2006). Job satisfaction among school psychologists: A meta-analysis. *School Psychology Quarterly, 21*(1), 77-90.

Vernon, A. (1998). *The Passport Program.* Champaign, IL: Research Press.

Walker, H. M., & Sprague, J. R. (1999). Longitudinal research and functional behavioral assessment issues. *Behavioral Disorders, 24,* 335–337.

Ward, S. B. (2001). Intern supervision in school psychology: Practice and process of field-based and university supervisors. *School Psychology International, 22,* 269–84.

Webster-Stratton, C., & Reid, M. J. (2003). The incredible years parents, teachers, and children training series. In A. E. Kazdin & J. R. Weisz (Eds.), *Evidence-based psychotherapies for children and adolescents* (pp. 224–240). New York: Guilford Press.

Wechsler, D. (1949). *The Wechsler Intelligence Scale for Children.* New York: Psychological Corporation.

Wechsler, D. (1955). *The Wechsler Adult Intelligence Scale.* New York: Psychological Corporation.

Wechsler, D. (1997). *Wechsler Adult Intelligence Scale* (3rd ed.). San Antonio, TX: Psychological Corporation.

Wechsler, D. (2002a). *Wechsler Individual Achievement Test* (2nd ed.). San Antonio, TX: Psychological Corporation.

Wechsler, D. (2002b). *Wechsler Preschool and Primary Scale of Intelligence* (3rd ed.): *Administration and scoring manual.* San Antonio, TX: Psychological Corporation.

Wechsler, D. (2003). *Wechsler Intelligence Scale for Children* (4th ed.): *Technical and interpretive manual.* San Antonio, TX: Psychological Corporation.

Wertsch, J. V. (1985). *Vygotsky and the social formation of mind.* Cambridge, MA: Harvard University Press.

Wheeler, E., & Stomfay-Stitz, A. (2001). Working with families: Parents as partners in the peaceful classroom. *Childhood Education: Annual Theme, 77*(5), 318E–318F.

Willig, A. (1985). A meta-analysis of selected studies on the effectiveness of bilingual education. *Review of Education Research, 55,* 269–317.

Wnek, A. C., Klein, G., & Bracken, B. A. (2008). Professional development issues for school psychologists: What's hot, what's not in the United States. *School Psychology International, 29*(2), 145–160.

Wodrich, D. L., & Pfeiffer, S. I. (1989). *School psychology in medical settings* Hillsdale, NJ: Erlbaum.

Wood, D., Bruner, J. S., & Ross, G. (1976). The role of tutoring in problem solving. *Journal of Child Psychology and Psychiatry, 17*(2), 89–100.

Woodcock, R. W., McGrew, K. S., & Mather, N. (2001a). *Woodcock-Johnson III Tests of Cognitive Ability.* Itasca, IL: Riverside.

Woodcock, R. W., McGrew, K. S., & Mather, N. (2001b). *Woodcock-Johnson III Tests of Achievement.* Itasca, IL: Riverside.

Woody, R. H., LaVoie, J. C., & Epps, S. (1992). *School psychology: A developmental and social systems approach.* Needham Heights, MA: Allyn & Bacon.

Wright, M., & Mullan, F. (2006). Dyslexia and the Phono-Graphix reading programme. *Support for Learning, 21*(2), 77–84.

Young, B. A. (2002). *Public school student, staff and graduate counts by state: School year 2000–2001.* Washington, DC: National Center for Education Statistics.

Ylvisaker, M., Hartwick, P., & Stevens, M. (1991). School reentry following head injury: Managing the transition from hospital to school. *Journal of Head Trauma Rehabilitation, 6,* 10–22.

Zins, J. E., & Erchul, W. P. (2002). Best practices in school consultation. In A. Thomas, & J. Grimes (Eds.), *Best practices in school psychology* (4th ed., pp. 625–644). Bethesda, MD: National Association of School Psychologists.

Autism spectrum disorders—a group of disorders of varying severity characterized by difficulties in communication, social interaction, and behavioral deficits and excesses.

Behavior intervention plan (BIP)—takes the observations made in a functional behavioral assessment and turns them into a concrete plan of action for managing a student's behavior.

Cattell-Horn-Carroll Theory (CHC Theory)—a theory about the content and structure of human cognitive abilities that defines 10 broad stratum factors and over 70 narrow abilities. CHC theory is particularly relevant to school psychologists for psychoeducational assessment.

Curriculum-based assessment (CBA)—a method of systematically assessing a student's performance in the local curriculum.

Ecological-transactional model—a model of human behavior that forms the core conceptual base of school psychology. It posits that environmental factors that influence behavior interact in complex ways and that these interactions are transactional, meaning a child's behavior and development are influenced by the interactions between other developing individuals and a changing environment.

Evidence-based interventions (EBI)—a class of interventions that meets the criteria set by a professional group and that has research-based evidence of its effectiveness for addressing a particular problem.

Fixed battery—a set of predetermined assessment tests used for all psychoeducational referral concerns.

Flexible battery—a set of tests specifically chosen for a particular child based on the school psychologist's hypotheses.

Formative evaluation—using current student data to evaluate the quality of interventions and instructional support within the classroom, school, or district.

Functional behavioral assessment (FBA)—an assessment approach focused on interpersonal and learning behavior in the context of the local learning environment that is characterized by breaking down complex behavior to antecedents, behaviors, and consequences.

Individual Education Program (IEP)—an individualized educational plan that is designed to meet the unique educational needs of one child, as defined by federal regulations.

Individuals with Disabilities Education Improvement Act (IDEA)—a law ensuring a free, appropriate public education to children with disabilities throughout the nation.

NASP—National Association of School Psychologists, the largest professional organization representing school psychologists.

Omnibus measures—questionnaires that assess a wide range of behavior and affect that cover desirable and nondesirable dimensions. Modern measures often permit multiple raters (e.g., parents and teachers) to comment on the child's strengths and weaknesses

Rational emotive behavior therapy (REBT)—a type of psychotherapy that focuses on resolving emotional and behavioral problems and disturbances. The underlying premise is that an individual's thoughts about a problem, as opposed to the problem itself, determine the extent of the disturbance.

Reflective practice—thoughtfully considering one's own experiences in applying knowledge to practice; novices are typically coached by professionals in the discipline. It is part of ongoing professional learning.

Reliability—describes the consistency of a measure, the degree to which a test measures the same way each time it is used. It is an indication of the amount of measurement error expected in the use of a test for a particular group of individuals; higher reliability indicates lower measurement error. Reliable measures generate scores that are repeatable.

Response-to-intervention (RTI)—a framework for providing tiered instructional services for youth; it can assist with the identification of students with learning disabilities.

Validity—the degree to which evidence and theory support the interpretations of test scores; it is a property of measurement that determines the extent to which a measurement method measures what was intended.

Wicked problem—a problem that has incomplete, contradictory, and changing parameters in a context of complex interdependencies.

INDEX

Note: Page number followed by "*t*" denote tables.

ABOUT THE AUTHORS

Rosemary Flanagan, PhD, ABPP is an associate professor in the School Psychology Program at Touro College, New York. Previously she was a full-time faculty member and director of the school psychology program at the Gordon F. Derner Institute for Advanced Psychological Studies at Adelphi University, Garden City, New York. Prior to coming to Adelphi, she was a practicing school psychologist for 18 years, while serving as adjunct faculty at St. John's and Hofstra Universities. She has taught personality assessment for more than 15 years and has over 20 publications on assessment, intervention, and professional issues in school psychology. She is a member of the editorial board of *Psychology in the Schools* and has served as a co-guest editor of special issues of the journal. She is a Fellow of the American Academy of School Psychology and the Society for Personality Assessment, an Associate Fellow of the Albert Ellis Institute, and a Diplomate of the American Board of Professional Psychology (ABPP). She has served ABPP in numerous capacities, having been president of the American Board of School Psychology and a member of the ABPP Board of Trustees. She maintains an independent practice of psychology. She received her PhD in clinical and school psychology from Hofstra University.

Jeffrey A. Miller, PhD, ABPP, is professor of school psychology at Duquesne University. He is a Fellow and past president of the American Academy of School Psychology. He also serves on the board of the American Board of School Psychology and is vice-president of the Council of Specialties in Professional Psychology. He has published over 30 books, book chapters, and refereed journal articles. He is on the editorial boards of the *Journal of Psychoeducational Assessment* and the *Journal of Applied School Psychology*. His research focuses on the translation of neuropsychological knowledge to improve teaching and learning and professional issues in school psychology.